A Clinical Guide To Occlusion

A Clinical Guide to Occlusion

S J Davies
Lecturer in Dental Practice, University Dental Hospital of Manchester
General Dental Practitioner, Stockport

R J M Gray
Honorary Fellow, University Dental Hospital of Manchester
General Dental Practitioner, Altrincham

Specialist Contributors

J A James
Lecturer in Oral Pathology and Periodontics, University Dental Hospital of Manchester

G J Linden
Reader in Periodontolgy, School of Dentistry, Queens University, Belfast

I C Mackie
Senior Lecturer/Honorary Consultant, Unit of Paediatric Dentistry, University Dental Hospital of Manchester

J F McCord
Professor of Restorative Dentistry, Unit of Prosthodontics, University Dental Hospital of Manchester

K D O'Brien
Professor of Orthodontics, University Dental Hospital of Manchester

J E Qualtrough
Senior Lecturer and Honorary Consultant in Restorative Dentistry, University Dental Hospital of Manchester

P J Sandler
Consultant Orthodontist, Royal Hospital, Callow, Chesterfield

P W Smith
Lecturer and Honorary Consultant in Restorative Dentistry, University Dental Hospital of Manchester

S A Whitehead
Consultant in Restorative Dentistry, Carlisle

M P J Young
Research Associate, University Dental Hospital of Manchester
BUPA Hospital, Manchester

2002
Published by the British Dental Association
64 Wimpole Street, London, W1G 8YS

Preface

I would like to thank Mike Grace, Stephen Hancocks and Peter Fyne at the *British Dental Journal* for their encouragement, advice and hard work in the preparation of this work.

Gordon Lucas, Andrew Morris, Ray Richmond, Ziad Al-Ani, Alan Jack, Tracy Davenport, Janine Jacobs, Clive Attack and Paul Hine have all helped with the production of models, diagrams or photographs.

Alan Quayle is a constant source of encouragement and above all without the support, guidance and expertise of my co-author Robin Gray this work would never have been completed.

Finally I would like to thank my wife, who has no interest in occlusion, for her sacrifice and understanding during the time that this project has taken to complete.

Dedication

This book is dedicated to two groups of dentists.

Firstly to the specialists listed on page iii, who welcomed the challenge of viewing their specialities from an occlusal perspective and without whose expertise, academic discipline and open mindedness this work would have been impossible.

Secondly, it is dedicated to the ever increasing number of dentists who wish to 'go the extra mile' of incorporating good occlusal practice into their everyday work.

Stephen Davies

© **British Dental Journal 2002**

Reprinted 2003, 2006

ISBN 0 904588 68 8

Printed and bound by Dennis Barber Limited, Lowestoft, Suffolk

Contents

A clinical guide to occlusion: an introduction

Robert G. Jagger,[1]

Dental undergraduates are usually taught the theoretical basis of occlusion and are left in no doubt that occlusion is important. The increasingly congested dental curriculum however means that they usually have very limited practical clinical experience and this is true of occlusal problems in particular.

The newly qualified dentist then often suffers a degree of confusion and uncertainty. He or she is involved every day in treatments that affect the dental occlusion — but what exactly is an occlusal interference? What sort of occlusion is necessary for a new prosthesis? What are the consequences of malocclusions and occlusal interferences? Are occlusal treatments necessary and if so when and how should they be carried out?

Attending postgraduate courses on occlusion can often help the situation. The confusion can be compounded though, when different 'experts' give contradictory information. Often clinical opinions are presented as facts or 'rules'. This is sometimes taken to extremes by some dentists who claim that all manner of disorders can be caused by occlusal interferences.

The authors of this series have confronted the dilemma head-on and written a series of ten articles with the aim of providing a working guide for the practical dentist. They have produced this series of articles based on best current evidence. No exaggerated or unsubstantiated claims are made about the consequences of occlusal interferences nor about the benefits of occlusal treatments.

This series is aimed at practical dentists but is not a 'how-to-do' handbook. It is designed to provide a working philosophy that is in line with contemporary good practice to be used in everyday clinical practice. Recommendations are supported by evidence from clinical research wherever possible. The authors however acknowledge the need sometimes to draw on the body of clinical experience and perceived wisdom and sensible reasons are given for recommendations if clinical evidence is lacking.

Each article begins with clearly stated aims and concludes with a short list of guidelines for good clinical practice, directly related to the aims. Successive chapters then build on the preceding chapters, each adding in turn to the list of guidelines. This results, at the end of the series of articles, in a comprehensive list that is the 'Guidelines of good clinical practice'.

The series begins with two chapters that describe the masticatory system and how to examine temporomandibular joints, muscles of mastication and the dental occlusion.

The majority of the remaining articles discuss occlusion in relation to restorative dentistry, including operative dentistry, fixed and removable prosthetics, dental implants and periodontology. The conformative and re-organisation approaches form the foundations of the prosthetic articles and techniques of occlusal reconstruction appropriate to different prostheses are thoroughly described

Two other articles include occlusal considerations in orthodontics and paediatric dentistry and a final article deals with tooth surface loss.

Each article can stand alone and includes several important references but is designed to complement the other articles eventually producing the set of practical guidelines.

The authors have produced a novel approach to the subject, and dentists should find the step-by-step method logical and convenient and above all of practical value. The series should help dispel some myths about occlusion and help dentists treat their patients at the same time as recognising that there is more to learn.

[1]Senior Lecturer/Consultant in Restorative Dentistry, Department of Adult Dental Health, Dental School, Heath Park, Cardiff, CF14 4XY
email: Jagger@Cardiff.ac.uk

1

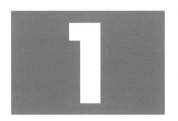

What is occlusion?

S. Davies,[1] and R. J. M. Gray,[2]

The aim of this series of papers is to explore the role of occlusion in dental practice. The range of opinion in the dental profession as to the importance of occlusion is enormous.[1] It is very important that the profession in general and practising dentists in particular have a balanced view of occlusion. This is more important than every patient having a balanced occlusion. The fact that the study of occlusion is characterised by extremes makes it confusing and possibly difficult for individual dentists to find a philosophy which is in line with contemporary good practice supported by evidence from practice-based research.

[1]*GDP, 73 Buxton Rd, High Lane, Stockport SK6 8DR; P/T Lecturer in Dental Practice, University Dental Hospital of Manchester, Higher Cambridge St., Manchester M15 6FH; [2]Honorary Fellow, University Dental Hospital of Manchester, Higher Cambridge St., Manchester M15 6FH *Correspondence to : Stephen Davies, 73 Buxton Rd, High Lane, Stockport SK6 8DR email: stephen.j.davies@man.ac.uk

In this part, we will discuss:
- **What 'occlusion' is**
- **Why occlusion is important**
- **The significance of 'ideal occlusion'**

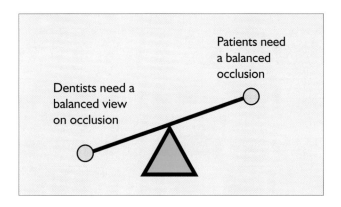

At one end of the spectrum are dentists who believe that they can go through their working lives with scant regard for their patients' occlusion. They seem to believe that essentially they can conduct their practice ignoring the occlusal consequences of the treatments that they perform daily. Whereas all dentists know of the importance of the good marginal adaptation of their restoration to the health of the adjoining dental and periodontal tissues, some dentists do not appreciate the potential consequences of poor occlusal contact to the opposing teeth and their supporting structures. This is bizarre given the fact that very few dental treatments do not involve the occlusal surfaces of teeth.

Conversely there is a body of opinion that considers occlusion to be such a central pillar in our working lives, and to be of such systemic import to the well being of our patients, that 'occlusion' takes on an almost mystic importance and attracts a cult like devotion (Fig. 1). This can lead some dentists to advocate occlusion as being the key to resolving or preventing a range of disorders far removed from the mas-

ticatory system, for example prolapsed lumbar discs. Often such enthusiastic fervour is associated with a didactic prescription of 'occlusal rules' which must be adhered to in the treatment of *every* patient.

The danger is that both of these approaches leads to inappropriate levels of patient care; patients suffer through either over or under treatment.

It is not surprising that these two extreme views co-exist so easily within a thinking profession because the one appears to provide the justification for the other. The 'occlusion doesn't matter' group probably justify their reluctance to become 'involved in occlusion' on the grounds of what they perceive to be the exaggerated and unsubstantiated claims of the group who believe occlusion to be the central pillar of holistic care. This congregation of opinion in turn may be so frustrated by the apparent disregard of the study of occlusion that they are led to 'gild the lily' by overstating the importance of occlusion and then in the absence of what they perceive to be an inability 'to see the obvious' they go on to lay down rules.

It is the objective of this series of papers to explore the role of occlusion in dental practice in a manner based on reason. There is good and bad practice in occlusion as in other aspects of clinical dentistry: we wish, therefore, to establish the concept of Good Occlusal Practice, which is applicable to all disciplines in dentistry.

Guidelines of good occlusal practice

These should be guidelines not rules.

All patients are different, reacting to similar stimuli in different ways. So the detail of a patient's individual needs can and should be left to the individual clinician. These Guidelines of Good Occlusal Practice should appear to be common sense and, upon reflextion, we hope that the reader will agree that they are obvious. We argue that any fog that has descended over this subject must be cleared, because no practising dentist can care well for their patients without having regard for good occlusal practice.

The importance of occlusion in dental practice

Occlusion can be defined very simply: it means the contacts between teeth.

Before describing the significance of the different ways in which occlusal contacts are made occlusion needs to be put into context.

The masticatory (or stomatognathic) system (Fig. 2) is generally considered to be made up of three parts: the Teeth, the Periodontal Tissues, and the Articulatory System.

It is a common criticism of dentists that our dental schools ignore the third part of the masticatory system, the articulatory system, in their teaching. It appears that dentists feel that their time at university did not prepare them adequately in this area; and this view seems to be the case worldwide. The undergraduate dental education must, however, by necessity

Fig. 1	It has been claimed without evidence that occlusion causes:

- Temporomandibular disorders
- Poor posture
- Excessive ear wax
- Speech defects
- Prolapse of lumbar disc

- Negative influence on the craniosacral mechanism
- Lack of beauty
- Reduced strength in Deltoid and Rectus Femoralis muscles

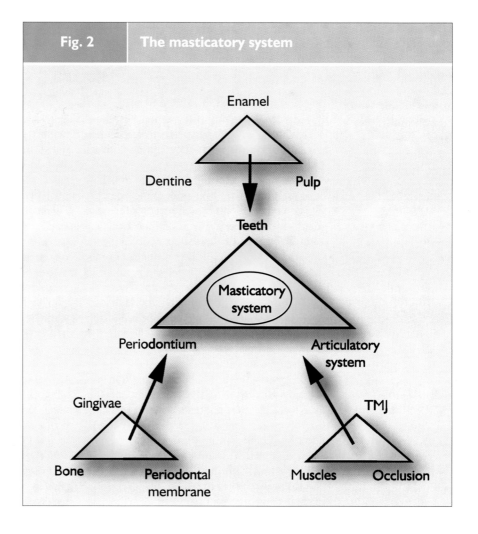

Fig. 2	The masticatory system

Enamel

Dentine · Pulp

Teeth

Masticatory system

Periodontium · Articulatory system

Gingivae · TMJ

Bone · Periodontal membrane · Muscles · Occlusion

concentrate initially on the first two parts of this triumvirate, because the dental schools must produce newly qualified dentists who are able to treat patients. Only once the dental undergraduate has an understanding of the diseases that affect the dental and periodontal tissues (parts 1 and 2 of the masticatory system) can the schools start to allow the student to treat patients. So there is justification for the study of the articulatory system being considered to be the third area of study from a chronological point of view. But because of the inescapable fact that almost all dental treatment has an occlusal consequence, it is wrong to consider the study of the articulatory system to be less important than the first two parts of the masticatory system. Given the increasing quantity of knowledge to be amassed in the modern undergraduate course, it may be that those responsible for setting the dental undergraduate curriculum will not be able to cover the articulatory system as they would wish. Now that there is a universal acceptance of the need for continuing education, it may be more realistic to consider a comprehensive study of the articulatory system as the first mandatory element of a post graduate dental education. But the articulatory system is the biomechanical environment in which dentists provide treatment. Although it maybe, by necessity, the last to be learnt it is not less important than the other parts of the masticatory system.

Is the articulatory system a true system?
(Fig. 3a, b)
A system is defined as: 'An assemblage that is connected or interdependent, so as to form a complex unity.' [OED] The articulatory system meets these criteria, so the answer to this question is: Yes.

In this system one can imagine the temporomandibular joints as the hinges, the masticatory muscles as the motors and the dental occlusion as the contacts (Fig. 3b).

When viewed in mechanical terms (Fig. 3b) it is clear that the elements of the articulatory system are inescapably connected. Furthermore, it can be argued that they are obviously *interdependent* because a change in any part will clearly affect the other two parts (Fig. 4a), but this effect will not necessarily be adverse.

The same sort of analysis of the interconnection within the masticatory system can be made (Fig. 4 b).

The importance of 'occlusion' in dental practice is based primarily upon the relationships that it has within these interconnected biomechanical systems. When one considers how almost all forms of dental treatment have a potential for causing occlusal change, the need to establish what constitutes good occlusal practice is overwhelming and obvious.

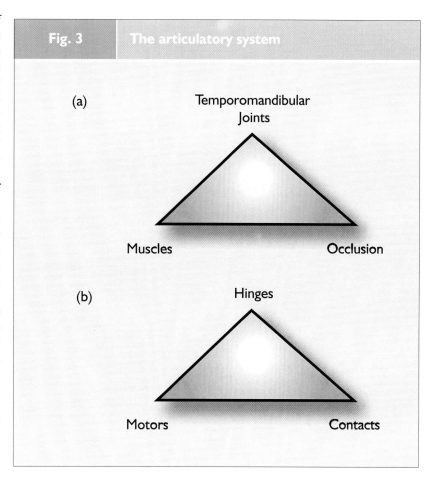

Fig. 3   The articulatory system

(a) Temporomandibular Joints / Muscles / Occlusion

(b) Hinges / Motors / Contacts

Analysis of occlusion
Having stated that occlusion simply means the contact between teeth, the concept can be further refined by defining those contacts between the teeth when the mandible is closed and stationary as the static occlusion, and those contacts between teeth when the mandible is moving relative to the maxilla as the dynamic occlusion.

Static occlusion
The first essential question when considering a patient's static occlusion is: 'Does centric occlusion occur in centric relation?'

This question will be clarified after defining terminology, which has been a 'red herring' and has been the cause of enormous and sometimes acrimonious debate. We also have preferred terms, but do not feel that they are important.

Centric Occlusion (CO) can be described as the occlusion the patient makes when they fit their teeth together in maximum intercuspation. Common synonyms for this are Intercuspation Position (ICP), Bite of Convenience or Habitual Bite. It is the occlusion that the patient nearly always makes when asked to close their teeth together, it is the 'bite' that is most easily recorded. It is how unarticulated models fit together. Finally, it should be remembered that it is the occlusion to which the patient is accustomed ie the habitual bite.

A clinical guide to occlusion

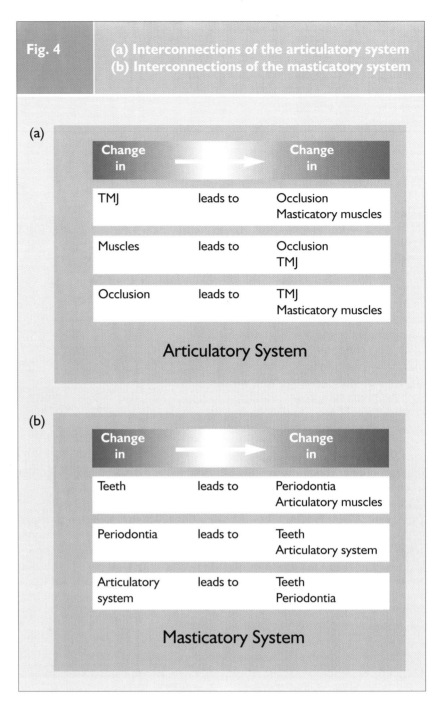

Fig. 4 (a) Interconnections of the articulatory system
(b) Interconnections of the masticatory system

(a)

Change in		Change in
TMJ	leads to	Occlusion Masticatory muscles
Muscles	leads to	Occlusion TMJ
Occlusion	leads to	TMJ Masticatory muscles

Articulatory System

(b)

Change in		Change in
Teeth	leads to	Periodontia Articulatory muscles
Periodontia	leads to	Teeth Articulatory system
Articulatory system	leads to	Teeth Periodontia

Masticatory System

> The word **'Centric'** is an adjective. It should only be used to qualify a noun. **Centric** *what?*

Centric Relation (CR) is not an occlusion at all. CR has nothing to do with teeth because it is the only 'centric' that is reproducible with or without teeth present. Centric Relation is a jaw relationship: it describes a conceptual relationship between the maxilla and mandible. All attempts to lay down rigid definitions of centric relation are plagued by the fundamental difficulty that there is no sure or easy way of proving that the locating criteria have been achieved.

Centric Relation has been described in three different ways: anatomically, conceptually,[2] and geometrically.

Anatomical
Centric Relation can be described as the position of the mandible to the maxilla, with the intra-articular disc in place, when the head of the condyle is against the most superior part of the distal facing incline of the glenoid fossa. This can be paraphrased as uppermost and foremost (Fig. 5).

This is subject to debate. Some clinicians prefer the idea that centric relation occurs in an 'uppermost and midmost' position within the glenoid fossa; whereas very few people now support the idea that it is in an 'uppermost and rearmost' position. There is support for the uppermost and foremost hypothesis from a study of anatomy: the bone and fibrous articulatory surfaces are thickest in the anterior aspect of the head of the condyle and the most superior aspect of the articular eminence of the glenoid fossa. This is, however, of only academic interest and not of clinical significance as there is no reliable simple means of determining the exact

6

position of the head of the condyle within the glenoid fossa.

Conceptual

Centric relation can be described as that position of the mandible relative to the maxilla, with the articular disc in place, when the muscles that support the mandible are at their most relaxed and least strained position. This description is pertinent to an understanding of 'ideal occlusion'. This definition supports the concept of a 'qualitative' relationship between a jaw position and another element of the articulatory system.

Geometrical

Centric Relation can be described 'as the position of the mandible relative to the maxilla, with the intra-articular disc in place, when the head of the condyle is in terminal hinge axis'.

In order to understand what this frequently used definition means it is easier, initially, to think about one side of the mandible only. The mandible opens by firstly a rotation of the condyle and then a translation which is downwards and forwards. Therefore, when the mandible closes the the terminal closure is purely rotational. At this phase of closure the mandible is describing a simple arc, because the centre of its rotation is stationary. This provides the 'terminal hinge point' (of rotation) of one side of the mandible; but because the mandible is one bone with two connected sides these two terminal hinge points are connected by an imaginary line: *the terminal hinge axis*. This axis is, therefore, envisaged by imagining the stationary, centres of rotation of each condyle whilst the mandible is moving only in the rotational phase of movement. It is the fact that the mandible is describing this simple arc, when the heads of condyle are in the terminal hinge axis which is of the most clinical significance. This will be discussed later, when the techniques for finding centric relation are presented.

Significance of Centric Relation

There may be arguments about the exact position of centric relation and on how that position is clinically best found. There is, however, a broad agreement between dentists who have studied this subject that there exists a *reproducible* position of the mandible relative to the maxilla, and that this position is reproducible irrespective of the guidance that the occlusal surfaces of the teeth may provide. Patients with no teeth still have a centric relation. Furthermore there is inter- and intra-operator reliability in finding it.

'Freedom in centric'

Another aspect of the static occlusion is the presence or absence of 'freedom in centric', this is also known as 'long centric'.

As previously stated the word centric is an

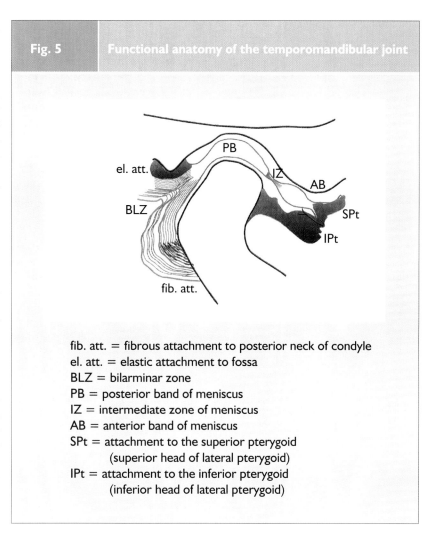

| Fig. 5 | Functional anatomy of the temporomandibular joint |

fib. att. = fibrous attachment to posterior neck of condyle
el. att. = elastic attachment to fossa
BLZ = bilarminar zone
PB = posterior band of meniscus
IZ = intermediate zone of meniscus
AB = anterior band of meniscus
SPt = attachment to the superior pterygoid
 (superior head of lateral pterygoid)
IPt = attachment to the inferior pterygoid
 (inferior head of lateral pterygoid)

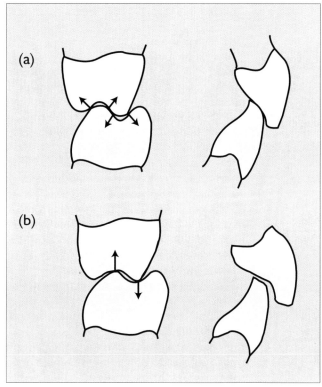

Fig.6
(a) No freedom in centric occlusion
(b) Freedom in centric occlusion

adjective and so strictly it should never be used without a defining noun. So this long established term would better read: Freedom in centric occlusion or long centric occlusion. Freedom in centric occlusion occurs when the mandible is able to move anteriorly for a short distance in the same horizontal and sagittal plane while maintaining tooth contact (Fig. 6b). Alternatively there will be no freedom in centric occlusion if either the front teeth or the posterior occlusion do not allow this horizontal movement (Fig. 6a).

An easier way of imagining Freedom in Centric Occlusion is to state that if the front teeth hit together as hard or harder than the back teeth, then there is no freedom in that centric occlusion. Two common examples of occlusions that may not have this freedom are firstly those which have an Angles Cl II div (ii) incisor relationship and secondly when anterior crowns have been provided with palatal surfaces which are too thick.

In Figure 6a, there is no freedom in centric occlusion as the occlusal contacts 'lock in' the mandible to the maxilla. Whereas in Figure 6b the mandible can move anteriorly, for a short distance, in the same sagital and horizontal plane.

Other aspects of the static occlusion that can be described are the extent of the posterior support, the Angle's classification of the incisor relationship together with measurement of the overbite and overjet, and the existence of any cross bites.

The answer to the question: 'Does Centric Occlusion occur in Centric Relation?' is therefore essential, because it describes the relationship of the mandible to the maxilla when the teeth fit together.

Dynamic occlusion

The dynamic occlusion refers to the occlusal contacts that are made whilst the mandible is moving relative to the maxilla. The mandible is moved by the muscles of mastication and the pathways along which it moves are determined not only by these muscles but also by two guidance systems.

The posterior guidance system of the mandible is provided by the temporomandibular joints. As the head of the condyle moves downwards and forwards the mandible is moving along a guidance pathway which is determined by the intra-articular disc and the articulatory surfaces of the glenoid fossa, all of which is enclosed in the joint capsule.

If teeth are touching during a protrusive or lateral movement of the mandible then those (touching) teeth are also providing guidance to mandibular movement. This is the anterior guidance and this is provided by *whichever* teeth touch during excentric movements of the mandible.

No matter how far back these teeth are they are anterior to the temporomandibular joints and so a patient with a severe anterior open bite would still always have anterior guidance of their mandible, it could, for instance be on the second molars. Therefore, despite the ambiguity of the word 'anterior' in the term anterior guidance, it does not mean that the anterior guidance of the mandible is always on the front teeth. This definition differs from that given in some restorative textbooks, when the term anterior guidance is used to describe *only* those anterior guidances which involve front teeth.

Anterior guidance may be further classified. 'Canine guidance' refers to a dynamic occlusion that occurs on the canines during a lateral excursion of the mandible. A canine protected occlusion refers to the fact that the canine guidance is the only dynamic occlusal contact during this excursive movement.

Group function. In this type of anterior guidance the contacts are shared between several teeth on the working side during a lateral excursion. To qualify for the term 'group function', the contacts would be towards the front of the mouth and the most anterior of the group would be the earliest and hardest contacts. This would contrast with a 'working side interference', which infers a heavy or early occlusal contact towards the back of the mouth during an excursive movement. A 'non working side interference' is an anterior guidance on the back teeth on the non working side during lateral excursion. The working side is the side of the mandible *towards* which the mandible is moving during a lateral excursion. The non working side is the side of the mandible *away* from which the mandible is moving. These terms can be confusing when considering the temporomandibular joints, because it is the TMJ on the non working side which is moving the most.

One reason why restorative textbooks define anterior guidance as being solely the dynamic occlusal contacts between the front teeth is that it is generally considered to be more ideal if the anterior guidance is on those front teeth. Furthermore, the fact that the word 'interference' is used to describe an occlusal contact between back teeth infers that this anterior guidance is less ideal than others. This introduces the concept of 'ideal occlusion' and this raises two important considerations:

1. If some occlusions are ideal, for what or for whom are they ideal?
2. If occlusal contact between back teeth is deemed a posterior interference with what is it interfering?

Ideal occlusion

Let us examine this concept and question whether it has any useful function in routine clinical dentistry.

> 'Does Centric Occlusion Occur in Centric Relation?' This is an essential question.

> **Ideal Occlusion**
> Q. Who or what is it ideal for?
>
> **Posterior Interference**
> Q. Who or what is it interfering with?

If two molars on the side from which the mandible is moving during an excursive movement can be deemed to provide a non working side interference, then what are they interfering with?

The posterior guidance of the mandible is provided by the temporomandibular joints. As the head of the condyle translates down the articular eminence of the joint on the non working side (which, paradoxically is the side that is moving the furthest) the mandible is being guided by this joint. If, as this is happening, a posterior maxillary and mandibular tooth hit against each other and because these two posterior teeth are close to the joint, then there is potential for the contact between these two teeth to influence or 'interfere' with the movement of the condyle within that joint. Contrast this with the situation, where the anterior guidance is provided not by posterior teeth which are close to the joint, but by front teeth which are further away; then the likelihood of 'interference' of condylar movement within the non-working side temporomandibular joint is less.

Anterior guidance, therefore, on back teeth, whilst still providing anterior guidance to the mandible, is described as a posterior interference because it may interfere with the posterior guidance system of the mandible, namely the temporomandibular joints. Posterior interferences are, therefore, considered to be a less ideal type of dynamic occlusion; and the term ideal relates to whether or not it is ideal for another part of the articulatory system: the temporomandibular joints (Fig. 7a). The anterior guidance provided by front teeth is potentially more ideal for the temporomandibular joints for the simple reason that it is further away from the temporomandibular joints. Consequently it can be argued that one aspect of the occlusion (anterior guidance) may or may not be ideal for another part of the articulatory system.

It is, also, potentially more ideal if the teeth fit together (centric occlusion), in a position of the mandible relative to the maxilla, with the disc in place, where the muscles supporting the mandible are at their most relaxed and least strained (conceptual description of centric relation). This establishes another criterion of the occlusion that can be considered ideal or not ideal for the other part of the articulatory system, namely the muscles of mastication (Fig. 7b).

Definition of ideal occlusion
This is given in established texts as:[3]

1 The coincidence of Centric Occlusion in Centric Relation (CO = CR), when there is freedom for the mandible to move slightly forwards from that occlusion in the same

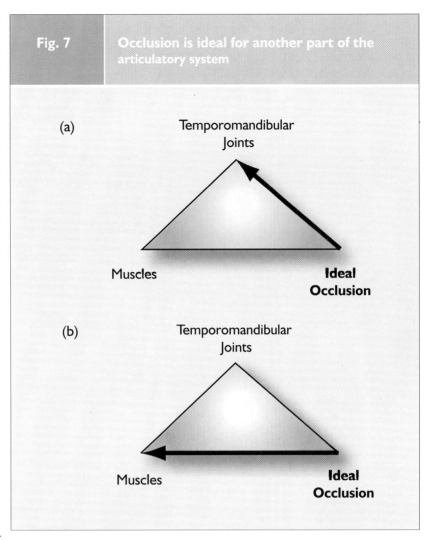

Fig. 7 Occlusion is ideal for another part of the articulatory system

(a) Temporomandibular Joints / Muscles / **Ideal Occlusion**

(b) Temporomandibular Joints / Muscles / **Ideal Occlusion**

sagittal and horizontal plane (Freedom in Centric Occlusion).

2 When the mandible moves there is immediate and lasting posterior disclusion (anterior guidance on front teeth)

It is presented in this section only after having considered for what or whom this type of occlusion is ideal, and the justification of why a particular type of occlusion could be considered as being potentially ideal for other parts of the articulatory system.

It is of paramount importance to appreciate that the term 'ideal occlusion' means something quite different from the term 'correct occlusion'. To state that an occlusion is correct or wrong betrays a mechanistic approach to the subject. Patients are not machines and an occlusion can only be judged on the reaction that it produces in the tissues of the system in which it inter-reacts. That reaction will be infinitely variable between individuals and will in some contexts (ie TMD pain) vary within an individual with time.

Guidelines of Good Occlusal Practice should be established because they offer the most prudent way in which to provide dental treatment to one part of the system whilst avoiding a potentially adverse reaction in another.

> There is no such thing as an intrinsically bad occlusal contact, only an **intolerable number of times** for that patient at that time in their life to function or parafunction on it

A clinical guide to occlusion

Fig. 8	Example of a record of a patient's occlusion, using ideal occlusion as the benchmark

Date 19/3/91	Occlusal record for	Robert Black 1 New St Old Town
	Skeletal 1 Angles 1	

Static occlusion

Does CO occur in CR? No

If not.. prem contact in CR? Roughly: Left molar

Exactly: Disto buccal cusp of lower left 8 against mesial marginal ridge of upper 7 and distal of upper left 6

Direction of slide from CR to CO: 3mm
Anterior slightly vertical and slightly to the left

Freedom in Centric Occlusion? No

Dynamic occlusion

		RHS	LHS
Non-working side interferences		17(FGC) v 48	No
Working side interferences		No	No
Crossover position	NWS Int	17 v 48	NO
	WS Int	No	No
Canine guidance		Yes (bridge 13)	No
Group function		No	No

Notes No tongue scalloping or cheek ridging
Tooth surface loss (anteriors) and history
of cuspal fracture at tooth 17

The importance of ideal occlusion as a concept

1. Pretreatment examination and records

The first and most important reason for defining ideal occlusion is that it gives a benchmark against which patients' occlusion can be measured. This needs to be done before, during and after dental treatment; especially in this increasingly litigious environment.

It is of paramount importance that dentists examine and record the pre-existing occlusion before providing treatment which involves changes to that occlusion. Study models would be a good way of doing this as long as they are mounted on an articulator in centric relation. At least the condylar guidance angles would also need to be correctly set so that the dynamic occlusion was recorded. This is not practicable for the vast majority of dentists. Alternatively and infinitely more easily notes can be made, which describe the patient's occlusion. These notes use criteria of ideal occlusion as a benchmark. To record an occlusion using only the criteria of Angle's classification is of very limited value, whereas to use the benchmark of ideal occlusion is considerable more informative (see Fig. 8).

2. Treatment of Pain Dysfunction Syndrome (PDS)

The second reason why ideal occlusion is an important concept is found in the long held view that the most important factor in the development of Pain Dysfunction Syndrome (PDS) is 'the individual patient's lack of adaptation to a less than ideal occlusion'. [4] This is not describing a causal relationship between a less than ideal occlusion and PDS, as different patients will have different thresholds of tolerances to occlusion, in fact the same patients have a different tolerance to their occlusions at different times. It is, however, the case that some patients, at some times, do react adversely to their less than ideal occlusions; and this can lead to pain and dysfunction.

For these patients the provision of an ideal

Force > Resistance

- Reduces tissue resistance
- Causes failure
- Promotes pain /dysfunction

occlusion is, therefore, one but by no means the only way of treating the condition. When an ideal occlusion is provided this should always be initially in a temporary and reversible way: that is a stabilisation splint. The indications for the provision of an ideal occlusion in the patient's natural dentition, for the treatment of PDS are very rare.

3. Conformative versus reorganised approach

In providing treatment with an occlusal element, one of the first questions to be decided in the treatment planning stage is whether the aim is to maintain the same occlusion during treatment. If the pretreatment occlusion is to be preserved, then the is described as 'conformative approach'.[5]

Some dental treatment, such as most major restorative and all orthodontic treatment, will however, inevitably change the patient's occlusion: this is known as the 'reorganised approach'. It is, therefore, prudent to design an occlusion that is more ideal and so potentially better tolerated by the patient's articulatory system.

Factors determining a patient's reaction to an occlusion

As stated an occlusion can only be judged as being good or bad in relation to the reaction it produces in the patient's tissues. In the same way that the danger of a substance can only be judged in relation to the concentration in which it occurs, a particular occlusal contact should be assessed in relation to the frequency at which it is made.

This is why bruxism is an important consideration in dentistry.

The 'occlusion' means the contacts between the teeth. The application of force from the muscles, through those occlusal contacts, results in load. Whether that load produces damage to tissues will depend on several factors:

1. The resistance of the tissues and/or restoration.
2. The magnitude of the force being applied.
3. The frequency of the force being applied.
4. The direction of the force being applied.
5. The number of contacts transmitting that force.

Risk management

The purpose of guidelines of good occlusal practice is to reduce the risk of damage occurring to the interrelated tissues of the masticatory system, and so increase the chances of a healthy function. This will reduce the chances of disease, mechanical failure and dysfunction or pain. Dentists can positively influence these factors as part of their care.

1 Smith B G N. Occlusion: 1. General Considerations. *Dent Update* 1991; 18: 141-145.
2 Gray R M J, Davies S J, Quayle A A. *Temporomandibular disorders: a clinical approach.* pp20 BDJ publications, 1995, 1997.
3 Ash M M, Ramfjord S P. *Occlusion* 4th ed. pp84-85. Philadelphia: Saunders, 1995.
4 Ramfjord S P, Ash M M. *Occlusion* 2nd ed. p178. Philadelphia: Saunders, 1971.
5 Wise M. Occlusion and restorative dentistry for the general dental practitioner. *Br Dent J* 1982; 152: 319-320.

Guidelines of good occlusal practice

1. The examination of the patient involves the teeth, periodontal tissues and the articulatory system.
2. There is no such thing as an intrinsically bad occlusal contact, only an intolerable number of times to parafunction on it.
3. The patient's occlusion should be recorded, before any treatment is started.

to be continued.....

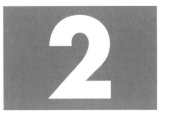

The examination and recording of the occlusion: why and how

S. J. Davies,[1] and R. J. M. Gray,[2]

Before presenting 'how' the examination and recording of the occlusion may be achieved, some attempt should be made to justify 'why' it is necessary. It may appear to be a strange way of justifying the need to examine the patient's occlusion, but this will initially involve a study of the influences of mandibular movements.

In this part, we will discuss:
- **How an understanding of mandibular locomotive systems compels dentists not to ignore occlusion**
- **How the occlusion can be simply and quickly examined and recorded**

[1]*GDP, 73 Buxton Rd, High Lane, Stockport SK6 8DR; P/T Lecturer in Dental Practice, University Dental Hospital of Manchester, Higher Cambridge St., Manchester M15 6FH; [2]Honorary Fellow, University Dental Hospital of Manchester, Higher Cambridge St., Manchester M15 6FH
*Correspondence to : Stephen Davies, 73 Buxton Rd, High Lane, Stockport SK6 8DR
email: stephen.j.davies@man.ac.uk

The mandible moves, relative to the maxilla, by virtue of two influences. Firstly, locomotive forces are provided by the muscles under the control of the nervous system: *neuromuscular control*. Secondly, there are two hard tissue *guidance systems:* these are the temporomandibular joints and the occlusal surfaces of the teeth.

Neuromuscular control

The muscles
Mandibular muscles
(The term mandibular muscles is preferable to masticatory muscles in the same way that 'leg muscles' is a more embracing term than 'walking muscles').

Within the articulatory system the muscles have been simply expressed as the 'motors'. Whereas it is the 'hard' occlusal surfaces of the teeth and articulatory surfaces of the bones which provide the guidances of mandibular movement, it is muscles which provide the locomotive force to move the mandible during function and parafunction. The muscles, which are joined to the mandible and are therefore responsible for its movement, are singularly and collectively immensely complicated motive entities.

It may be because anatomy was the first medical science, that the function of a muscle has historically been decided purely by an analysis of its origin and insertion. This is dangerously simplistic and has sometimes resulted in a mandibular muscle having been labelled as simply as an 'opening' or 'closing' muscle. It takes no account of the complex antagonistic and synergistic interrelations of muscle function, which are responsible for supplying the motive power of mandibular movement. Electromyographic recording when linked to either simple observation or sophisticated jaw tracking systems offers an enhanced understanding of the functions of the mandibular muscles. The lateral pterygoid muscle offers a good example of how the understanding of its function was enhanced by electromyography, beyond the simple anatomical assumptions previously held.[1]

Individual mandibular muscles
The masseter muscle
Anatomy: The masseter originates from the zygomatic arch, inserts into the outer surface of the angle of the mandible and comprises superficial, intermediate and deep parts.

Function: Its principal action is to elevate the mandible, so closing the jaws; it is also an accessory muscle in mandibular protrusion.

Parafunction: It is active in tooth clenching and is the most frequently affected muscle by this parafunctional habit.

The temporalis muscle
Anatomy: This is a large, fan shaped muscle arising from the lateral aspect of the skull in the temporal fossa and converges to a tendinous insertion, which, running below the zygomatic arch, inserts into both the coronoid process and anterior border of the ascending ramus of the mandible.

It is significant that the orientation of the muscle fibres varies greatly :

- The posterior fibres run almost horizontally forwards
- The anterior fibres run vertically.
- The intermediate fibres have varying degrees of orientation.

Function: The action of this muscle depends upon which fibres are contracting:

- The anterior fibres raise the mandible when the mouth is closing
- The horizontal posterior fibres retract the mandible. The horizontal fibres of the tem-

poralis muscle are the only muscle fibres that retract the mandible; no other muscle performs this function.

Parafunction: The temporalis muscle is the most frequently tender muscle in bruxists

Lateral pterygoid muscle
Anatomy: This is a muscle which has two heads and, it is now thought, two insertions. The smaller superior head arises predominantly from the infra-temporal surface of the greater wing of the sphenoid and inserts into the anterior part of the intra-articular disc and capsule, while the larger, inferior head arises from the lateral surface of the lateral pterygoid plate and inserts into the neck of the mandible just below the condyle.
Function: While it is accepted that there is some overlap of activity of the two heads, the superior pterygoid is predominantly active during clenching and is thought to stabilise the condyle disc assembly. The inferior pterygoid is active during mouth opening and draws the condyle and disc forwards and down the slope of the articular eminence.

Therefore, when both right and left pterygoid muscles act together, mouth opening and mandibular protrusion occurs, but when one muscle contracts the condyle on that side is drawn forwards and the mandible pivots around the opposing condyle and the chin, therefore, moves towards the opposite side.
Parafunction: This active/passive cycle is altered, however, in parafunction; when it has been demonstrated that there is an overall disruption of the pattern with both heads (or 'muscles' if superior and inferior bellies are considered to be separate muscles) showing a marked and simultaneous increase in activity. This can cause pain in the pre-auricular region. In addition, it may possibly lead to disc displacement, and the patient may develop TMJ clicking and locking.

The medial pterygoid muscle
Anatomy: The bulk of this muscle originates from the area between the two pterygoid plates; there is, however, a small, more superficial head arising from the maxillary tuberosity. These two heads fuse and the muscle passes posteriorly and laterally downwards to insert into the inner aspect of the angle of the mandible. The orientation of the fibres parallels that of the anterior fibres of the masseter muscle.
Function: The action of the medial pterygoid muscle is to elevate the mandible and it is also active during protrusion and lateral mandibular movement.
Parafunction: It is not a muscle that can reliably be palpated for tenderness, nor tested by resisted movement, and so its involvement in parafunction can only be surmised. It may

become hypertonic in patients who parafunction in extreme mandibular movement (eg the crossover position)

Digastric muscle
Anatomy: This muscle has two parts — the anterior and posterior bellies. They are connected by a tendon which passes through a fibrous loop on the upper border of the hyoid bone. The posterior belly arises from the mastoid notch and the anterior belly is inserted into the mandible near the symphysis. This insertion into the mandible qualifies it for inclusion as a 'mandibular muscle'.
Function: When the hyoid bone is fixed (by the infrahyoid muscles) the action of this muscle is to assist the lateral pterygoid muscle in opening the mouth. Its action is therefore to depress mandible. In the action of swallowing, the hyoid bone is raised by both right and left digastric muscles contracting together.
Parafunction: Tenderness in this muscle is frequently encountered in patients who brux or clench on their anterior teeth and manifests as pain behind the ascending ramus or under the body of the mandible.

Mylohyoid muscle
Anatomy: This thin sheet of muscle arises from the whole length of the mylohyoid line on the inner aspect of the mandible. The fibres meet in the median raphe, which inserts into the body of the hyoid bone. This muscle separates the submandibular and sublingual regions. Posteriorly the muscle has a free border.
Function: The action of this muscle is to raise the hyoid bone and the tongue during swallowing.

Suprahyoid, infrahyoid and cervical muscles
Function and parafunction: The reason why a brief consideration of the function and parafunction of these muscles should be discussed as part of the subject of occlusion is that claims are made that occlusion can have an effect on the wider musculo-skeletal system, even the lumbar spine. This supposition is based upon a consideration of head posture.

The hyoid bone is attached to the mandible by the suprahyoid muscles. The infrahyoid and suprahyoid muscles by stabilising the hyoid bone enable the suprahyoid muscles to be tangentially involved in mandibular movement. Head posture is also affected by the action of these muscles, as shown by the fact that the head moves slightly back as the mandible opens. Conversely, head posture could potentially affect the function and health of these muscles. This may provide an explanation for an association between head posture and myalgia of the head and neck muscles.

Similarly the cervical muscles are largely

responsible for head posture; and there may be an association between some TMD and symptoms of the cervical spine.

This hypothesis leads to the question, should dentists adjust the 'occlusion' to treat head and neck muscle pain?

It is right that dentists, together with other health professionals, constantly examine their understanding of the biomechanics of interlocking locomotive systems. It is obviously true that the occlusion of teeth is a part of this system, although a small part. But there is no evidence that a TMD follows the simple model of single cause, single diagnosis and single treatment and certainly there is no proof the occlusion is that single cause! We, therefore, feel that unless such a causal relationship is established, treatment to the teeth or permanent change of the position of the mandible is not indicated in pursuit of either a TMD or other musculo-skeletal disorder. In summary, 'thought, but not action' is appropriate.

Neural pathways

The mandible is controlled not only as a result of voluntary movement, but also by reflexes, most notably a jaw closing reflex and jaw opening reflex. The jaw-closing reflex protects the mandible and associated structures during violent whole body movement; it can result in damage to the teeth, especially if the occlusal contacts are not in the long axis of the root. The jaw opening reflex is to protect the teeth during sudden mastication of a hard object and to protect the lips, cheeks and tongue during mastication. These voluntary and involuntary movements are controlled by the central and autonomic nervous systems via sensory and motor nerves.

There is input to these systems from peripheral receptors and the higher centres, and also specific proprioceptors. These proprioceptors are not only situated in deep muscle, as in other human locomotive systems, but also in the periodontal ligaments. It is the presence of the periodontal proprioceptors which makes the articulatory system unique amongst human locomotive systems. No other locomotive system incorporates teeth which, because they are attached to proprioceptive receptors, means that if the movements within this locomotive system results in teeth touching (either in function or parafunction) then these proprioceptors are stimulated. As a consequence there is the potential for any change in a patient's occlusion, by routine dentistry, to 'be sensed' by the patient's nervous system. It is because of this consideration that dentists cannot ignore the effect of changing the occlusion when providing routine care.

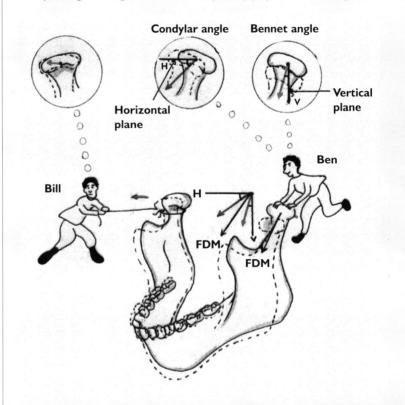

| Fig. I | Illustration of the direction of mandibular movement |

The direction of movement of the NWS condyle is forwards, downwards and medially (FDM). It is defined against the horizontal plane (H) by the condylar angle and against the vertical plane (V) by the Bennet angle.

This drawing is **not** designed to represent the muscles that are responsible for mandibular movement. Rather it is designed to illustrate how the NWS condyle moves forwards, downwards and medially; whereas the WS condyle undergoes an immediate non-progressive lateral movement. It is known as immediate side shift (ISS) or Bennet movement. The mandible moves **as if** Bill pulls it directly towards him, and Ben pushes it downwards, forwards and slightly towards Bill's side.

The guidance systems

There are two systems that provide hard guidance during mandibular movements. These are classified as the *posterior* and the *anterior* guidance systems but they are interrelated guidances and are part of one system. An understanding of them is important to dentists and relevant to this work, because occlusion provides one of them.

Posterior guidance

The temporomandibular joint is made up of the head of the condyle, the intra-articular disc and the glenoid fossa; and it provides the posterior guidance system of the mandible. During a lateral excursion of the mandible, the principle movement within the TMJs is on the non-working side (NWS).

The head of the condyle on the non-working side moves: forwards, downwards and medially.

- The angle of downwards movement is known as the 'condylar angle'
- The angle of medial movement is known as the 'Bennet angle'.

There is, however, a movement of the condyle on the working side as this is described as 'immediate side shift', or 'Bennet movement'. This movement is immediate, non progressive and lateral.

It is the mechanical consequence of the working side condyle being joined up to the non-working side condyle, whilst the latter is being pulled by muscles.

Figure 1 provides an illustration on mandibular movement during a right lateral excursion.

Anterior guidance

The anterior guidance system of the mandible is provided by which ever teeth touch during the excursive movements of the mandible, whilst teeth are in contact. These contacts are known as the dynamic occlusion.

Whilst it is generally considered to be more ideal if these contacts occur at the front of the mouth (ie as far away as possible from the posterior guidance system), it must surely be that even the back teeth may provide the anterior guidance of the mandible, because all teeth are anterior to the temporomandibular joints. The term 'anterior guidance' is often used in restorative textbooks to mean anterior guidance of the mandible which is exclusively on front teeth. This would be better described as 'ideal anterior guidance'. Ideal occlusion as a concept is described elsewhere in this work.

Relevance of a study of guidance systems to occlusion

The reason why dentists need to concern themselves with mandibular movements and the influences that control them is that most dental treatment involves the occlusal surfaces of teeth: that is to say that dentists inevitably are changing one of the guidance systems of mandibular movement.

There is little evidence to suggest that a change in occlusion will precipitate morphological changes within the joint. It would appear, therefore, that the most likely adaptation in the 'system' is that which can occur in the teeth and their supporting structures. These 'adaptations' are tooth wear, tooth movement and fracture.

Articulatory system: occlusal harmony?

How to determine what is an occlusion that conforms to the TMJ may appear to be an impossible question to answer; in reality the solution is very simple.

Firstly a competent examination of the whole of the articulatory system must be carried out. This will include the TMJs and the supporting muscles to determine whether there is any temporomandibular disorder present.

If there is a TMD present, then the first clinical decision to be taken, with the patient's involvement, will be whether or not to treat it before providing any other treatment.

Next, the patient's pretreatment occlusion must be examined, because, dependent upon the type and extent of the dental treatment necessary, the next essential treatment plan-

Fig. 2	Occlusal examination — question 1

Static occlusion

Does CO occur in CR?

If not.. prem contact in CR?   Roughly:
Exactly:

Direction of slide from CR to CO:

Fig. 3	Illustration of the relationship between the condyles moving when the mandible is in a terminal hinge axis and a 'perfect' arc as experienced during gentle bimanual manipulation

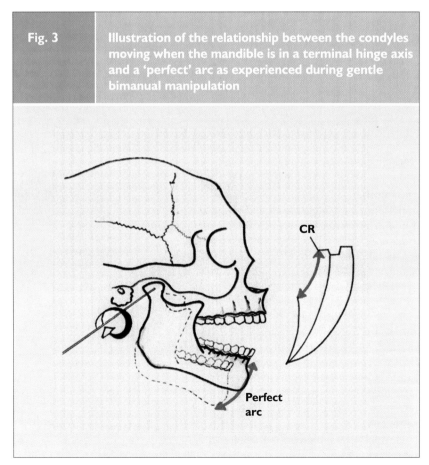

CR

Perfect arc

ning decision will be: 'can the treatment be provided without changing the patient's pre-existing occlusion?'

If it can, then the conformative approach is to be adopted. If it cannot, then it will be safer if the new occlusion is going to be more ideal rather than less ideal to the rest of the masticatory system than the pretreatment occlusion was. This is known as the 'reorganised approach'.

Either of these two approaches would constitute good occlusal practice. It would be bad occlusal practice accidentally or otherwise to make the occlusion a different or less ideal one.

This introduction has brought us to the conclusion that an examination of the patient's pre-treatment occlusion is essential.

Examination of the occlusion (Fig. 8)

Introduction
As stated in the previous section, the principle function of the concept of ideal occlusion in everyday dentistry is to provide a benchmark against which any patient's occlusal pattern can compared. This does not infer that the provision of an ideal occlusion is the treatment objective for that particular patient nor for patients in general.

The three question examination
Question 1. Does Centric Occlusion occur in Centric Relation? (Fig. 2)
Centric relation describes a relationship between the two jaws, it has nothing to do with teeth; it is not an occlusion. When the head of the condyle is moving purely in the rotational phase of its movement, then the mandible is in a *terminal hinge axis*. This concept provides one of the three pillars of the definition of centric relation that is given in the previous section. If the head of the condyle is the stationary centre about which the mandible is rotating, then the mandible, during this phase of movement will describe an arc. Whereas if the mandible is not in terminal hinge axis, then the head of the condyle will not be purely rotating, because there will be an element of translation; and as a consequence of the fact that the head of the condyle is, therefore, not stationary (in the antero-posterior plane) *the mandible will not describe an arc.*

Manipulation of patient to find the Centric Relation
It is the feeling that the patient's mandible is describing a perfect arc during manipulation that gives the experienced operator the confidence that the terminal hinge axis of the mandible (Fig. 3) has been found. It is certain that in reality the mandible is not describing a perfect arc because unlike on an articulator the condyle is never a perfect sphere and the

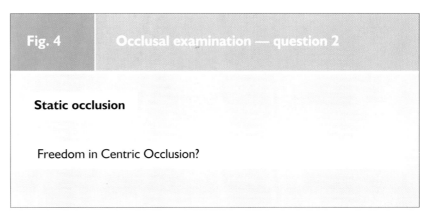

Fig. 4	Occlusal examination — question 2

Static occlusion

Freedom in Centric Occlusion?

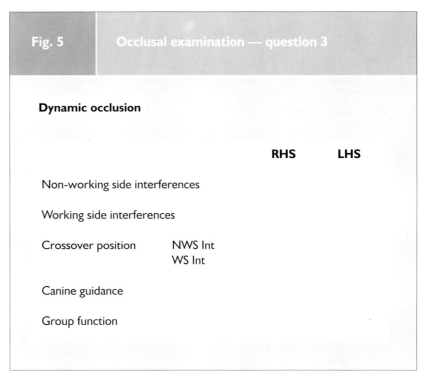

Fig. 5	Occlusal examination — question 3

Dynamic occlusion

	RHS	LHS
Non-working side interferences		
Working side interferences		
Crossover position — NWS Int		
WS Int		
Canine guidance		
Group function		

glenoid fossa is never a hemisphere. There is, however, one important test that provides confidence that Centric Relation has been found. This test is based upon the fact that because the Centric Relation is a jaw relationship not guided by teeth nor by the patient's muscles but by the operator arcing the mandible in its terminal hinge axis towards the maxilla, and that the end point of this arc *will be consistent.* The end point of this arc occurs when the first teeth touch and this is known as the premature contact in the Centric Relation. Centric Relation is the only 'Centric' which is consistent. It is the fact that the Centric Relation has been found to be consistent in any one patient irrespective of time or operator that makes it so significant as a concept. It may be that the end point of the closing arc of the mandible whilst it is in terminal hinge axis (Centric Relation) is not a premature contact but rather an even contact of all of the teeth (Maximum Intercuspation). In this case the Centric Relation and Centric Occlusion coincide. If, however, as is usually

A clinical guide to occlusion

Fig. 6   **How to find the Centric Relation**

- Operator seated comfortably
- Patient is supine, at elbow height
- Patient's neck extended slightly

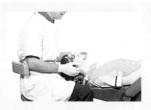

- Use both hands
- Thumbs over mental symphysis
- Fingers on the lower border of mandible, not sublingually

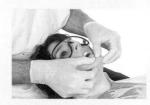

- Ask the patient to relax their jaw and let you *open* their mouth

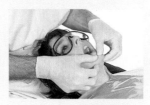

- Slowly and gently arc mandible up and down with minimum force
- Only the patient's mandible should be moving

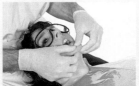 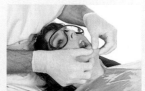 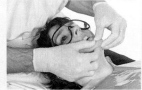

- Slowly increase the upward component of each arc, until premature contact is reached
- Ask the patient to put a finger in the air when they feel first contact

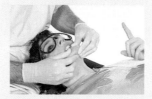

- Repeat at least three times
- Ask patient: It is the same each time?
- Ask patient to use raised finger to point where they feel first contact

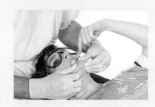

- Ask patient to squeeze teeth together from premature contact, so as to note the direction of slide

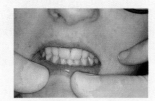

- With chairside assistance use articulating paper or foil to mark premature contact

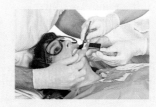

the case this ideal situation does not occur then the Centric Occlusion will not occur in Centric Relation. It will then be possible discover where the premature contact in Centric Relation is (Fig. 6). The positional difference between Centric Relation and Centric Occlusion can further be examined by noting the direction of slide of the mandible when the patient is asked to clench his or her teeth together whilst resting on the Centric Relation premature contact.

If Centric Relation (CR) and Centric Occlusion(CO) do not coincide, in many ways it would make more sense to describe the relationship between the jaws when the teeth are in Centric Occlusion, and not the other way round; but that is impossible to do because there are no landmarks on the jaws that can be examined whilst the patient is holding his or her teeth in Centric Occlusion. So the question has to be: ' Does CO occur in CR?'.

Question 2. Does the patient have Freedom in Centric Occlusion? (Fig. 4)

This investigation will answer the question: 'Is the patient's Centric Occlusion locked in?' This means when the patient is biting together normally, do his or her incisor teeth prevent those teeth moving slightly forward, or are they prevented from doing so (locked), by the fact that the lower incisor teeth heavily contact the palatal surfaces of the upper incisor teeth?

It can be examined by in one of three ways:

1. Marking the occlusal contacts and seeing if the anterior contacts are heavier than the posterior ones
2. Asking the patient to close together slowly and reporting which teeth hit first
3. Feeling for tremors on the upper incisor teeth with our finger nail whilst the patient repeatedly taps up into Centric Occlusion.

This was easier in the days before routine use of gloves.

Question 3. Where is the patient's Anterior Guidance? (Fig. 5)

It has already been discussed that the term 'anterior guidance' should not be taken to mean the guidance that is on the front teeth: it is the mandible that is being guided, by the temporomandibular joints (posterior guidance) and by the teeth (anterior guidance). Therefore, which ever teeth touch during excursive movements of the mandible provide the anterior guidance or the dynamic occlusion.

However, the benchmarch against which the patient's occlusion is measured is ideal occlusion (Fig. 7), and in an occlusion which is ideal for the rest of the articulatory system the anterior guidance is on the front teeth. When the anterior guidance is on the back teeth the terminology used is posterior interference. This may be either on the working or non-working side. If interferences are present then they may extend beyond the crossover position. If there are no posterior interferences, then the anterior guidance will be on the front teeth, and this is described as being either 'canine guidance' (where the contact between the upper and lower teeth during an excursive movement of the mandible is against the upper canine and then eventually on the upper central incisors); or it is described as a 'group function' where the anterior guidance is on several teeth. In a group function these contacting teeth are usually the canines and first and second premolars; the more anterior teeth of the group should provide the earlier and harder contacts, otherwise the contact could be considered as a working side interference.

Recording of the occlusion

It is essential to have a good record of the patient's occlusion if any treatment is to be provided that may have the potential for changing the occlusion. Even if no treatment is envisaged a complete examination of the patient should include the articulatory system of which the occlusion is one of key elements. Just as there are protocols of recording baseline measurements in periodontal and dental disease, there is a need to establish easy and universally reproducible ways of recording the patient's occlusion.

In addition, records are essential for medicolegal reasons.

These records can be either two or three dimensional.

1. Two dimensional records of the patient's occlusion

In the main, these rely on marking the static and dynamic occlusal contacts between the teeth and then describing those marks in writing, by diagram or by photograph. In addition to this use of articulating paper or foil to mark the contacts, floss or shimstock can be used to determine whether there is a contact ('pull through' test). The T-scan uses a computer program to analyse the relative hardness of the contacts between the teeth.

With the exception of the T-scan all these two dimensional techniques have the advantage that they are means of determining the occlusal contacts between the actual teeth. They have the disadvantage that is inherent in a two dimensional record of a three dimensional entity.

2. Three dimensional record of the patient's occlusion

This, of course, means study models. They have the advantage of being a permanent *copy* of the patient's occlusion, but the production

Fig. 7	How to examine anterior guidance

- Finding whether there are **Non working side** interferences, by trying 'a pull out'

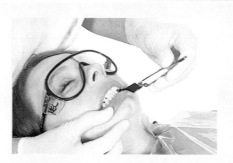

- During this right lateral excursion, there is a NWS interference between UL6 (26) and LL7 (37)

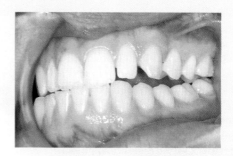

- Examining for the existence of **working side interferences** by marking the contact between the teeth during a slide to the working side (as illustrated)
- Next mark the centric occlusion stops in a different colour (not illustrated)

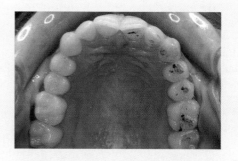

- Example of canine guidance

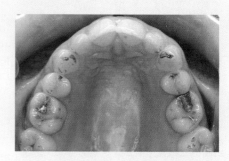

- Example of a group function

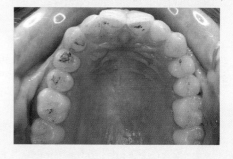

of this copy immediately introduces a host of potential errors. The impressions have to be accurate, the models from those impressions must not only be perfectly cast but also accurately related to each other in a static and dynamic occlusion. This depends not only upon face bows and articulators, but also on the correct use of a range of impression, registration and casting materials.

Discussion

Study models must be accurate otherwise they might as well not exist; so they need to be verified against either the patient at a check visit or against a second record which could be a simple two dimensional record of the patient's occlusion.

It is therefore the authors' contention that there is a need for a simple reliable two dimensional record of the patient's occlusion and that such a record would be very useful. Consequently these techniques will be illustrated in next section. The advantage of a two dimensional record of the occlusion is that it is not dependent upon a bite registration material, which may introduce error in the model mounting.[2]

Technique

Articulating paper or foil

If the intention is to mark the occlusal surface of a tooth in order to indicate the position of a contact as opposed to simply discovering whether there is such a contact (shimstock or floss), then a medium to retain some ink needs to be used. It may be double or single sided, but it must be thin and dry (Fig. 9).

At least two colours will be needed. Firstly so that the occlusal contacts in the static and dynamic occlusions can be differentiated; and secondly, so that in operative dentistry the occlusion pre- and post-treatment can be compared.

Articulators

Articulators are not essential. Their use is not a guarantee of success or of an easy life. Articulators are a very useful tool if the dentist wishes to go in the direction of reproducing the way in which the patient's jaws move one against another. This is valuable information as it assists in the accurate recording of the dynamic occlusion. The nearer a particular articulator can reproduce the patient's movements, the closer it will be possible to construct occlusal schemes that predictably conform to the dentist's objectives, whatever they may be.

In deciding which articulator to use, it is important to ask the question, 'What movements of the mandible do I wish to reproduce, for this patient at this time?'

The key point about this approach is that it

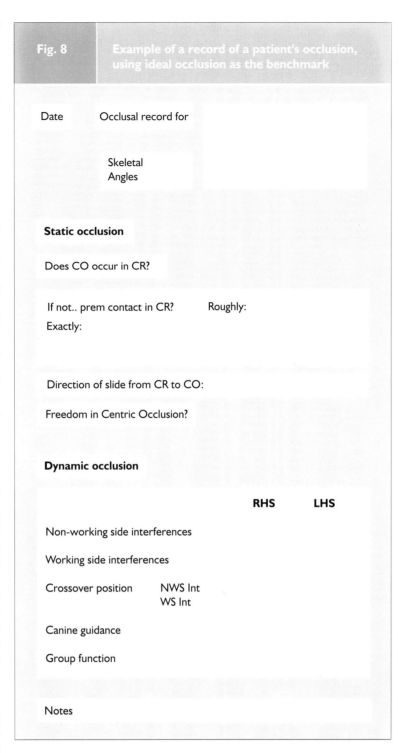

Fig. 8   Example of a record of a patient's occlusion, using ideal occlusion as the benchmark

Date   Occlusal record for

         Skeletal
         Angles

Static occlusion

Does CO occur in CR?

If not.. prem contact in CR?   Roughly:
Exactly:

Direction of slide from CR to CO:

Freedom in Centric Occlusion?

Dynamic occlusion

                           RHS   LHS

Non-working side interferences

Working side interferences

Crossover position   NWS Int
                      WS Int

Canine guidance

Group function

Notes

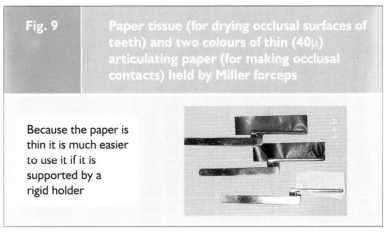

Fig. 9   Paper tissue (for drying occlusal surfaces of teeth) and two colours of thin (40μ) articulating paper (for making occlusal contacts) held by Miller forceps

Because the paper is thin it is much easier to use it if it is supported by a rigid holder

A clinical guide to occlusion

1 Juniper R P. Temporomandibular joint dysfunction; a theory based upon electromyographic studies of the lateral pterygoid muscle. *Br J Oral Maxillofac Surg* 1984; **22**: 1-8.
2 Walls A W G, Wassell R W, Steele J G. A comparison of two methods for locating the intercuspal position (ICP) whilst mounting casts on an articulator. *J Oral Rehab* 1991; **18**: 43-48
3 Cabot L B. Using articulators to enhance clinical practice. *Br Dent J* 1998; **184**: 272-276.

determines the level of predictability at which the dentist and technician wish to operate. If, as often is the case a dentist and technician are not going to operate with very sophisticated articulators, it does not mean that success is denied to them. It simply means that when checking the occlusion of the restoration it is more likely that adjustment will be necessary. Similarly, if a dentist and technician are operating with sophisticated articulation, it does not remove from the dentist the responsibility of checking the occlusion of the restoration at the fit appointment. A comprehensive overview of articulators can be found elsewhere.[3]

Facebows

A facebow is a device which enables the maxillary arch to be spatially related to various anatomical landmarks on the patient's face which assists in mounting the maxillary cast within the articulator. The most important consequence of this is that the maxillary cast (in the articulator it is the maxillary member which moves) will bear a similar relationship to the hinges of the articulator as the patient's TMJs does to his or her maxilla, and so to the mandible when a bite registration is used. This matters if the articulator is going to be used for anything other that the static occlusion in centric occlusion.

Guidelines for good occlusal practice

1. The examination of the patient involves the teeth, periodontal tissues and the articulatory system.
2. There is no such thing as an intrinsically bad occlusal contact, only an intolerable number of times to parafunction on it.
3. The patient's occlusion should be recorded, before any treatment is started.
4. **Compare the patient's occlusion against the benchmark of ideal occlusion.**
5. **A simple, two dimensional means of recording the patient's occlusion before, during and after treatment is an aid to good occlusal practice.**

Good occlusal practice in simple restorative dentistry

S. J. Davies,[1] R. J. M. Gray,[2] and P. W. Smith,[3]

Many theories and philosophies of occlusion have been developed.[1-12] The difficulty in scientifically validating the various approaches to providing an occlusion is that an 'occlusion' can only be judged against the reaction it may or may not produce in a tissue system (eg dental, alveolar, periodontal or articulatory). Because of this, the various theories and philosophies are essentially untested and so lack the scientific validity necessary to make them 'rules'. Often authors will present their own firmly held opinions as 'rules'. This does not mean that these approaches are to be ignored; they are, after all, the distillation of the clinical experience of many different operators over many years. But they are empirical.

In developing these guidelines the authors have unashamedly drawn on this body of perceived wisdom, but we would also like to involve and challenge the reader by asking basic questions, and by applying a common sense approach to a subject that can be submerged under a sea of dictate and dogma.

In this part, we will discuss:
- **The 'conformative approach' to restorative dentistry**
- **Some techniques for achieving this goal**
- **Can and should the occlusion be improved within the conformative approach?**

[1*]*GDP, 73 Buxton Rd, High Lane, Stockport SK6 8DR; P/T Lecturer in Dental Practice, University Dental Hospital of Manchester, Higher Cambridge Street, Manchester M15 6FH* [2]*Honorary Fellow, University Dental Hospital of Manchester, Higher Cambridge Street, Manchester M15 6FH* [3]*Lecturer/Honorary Consultant in Restorative Dentistry, University Dental Hospital of Manchester M15 6FH*
Correspondence to : Stephen Davies email: stephen.j.davies@man.ac.uk

Discussion

Does occlusion matter in simple restorative dentistry?

It is easy to justify a chapter on restorative dentistry in a book on occlusion. Dentists are constantly involved in the management of their patients' occlusion during routine restorative dental procedures. This is because the occlusal surfaces of the teeth are usually involved in the provision of restorations. The significance of this obvious statement lies both in the relationship that the occlusion has within the articulatory system and the effect that trauma from the occlusion may have on the tooth, and its periodontal support. All dentists wish to avoid these problems; in reality dentists want predictable success for their patients and themselves.

Successful occlusal management leads to: predictable fitting of restorations and prostheses, longevity and absence of iatrogenic problems, patient comfort and occlusal stability.

The starting point: examination

It is a general principle in medicine that before treatment is provided a careful clinical examination is carried out. Dentistry generally holds to this principle, but with perhaps one exemption. Most dentists were not taught at dental school to examine and record the pre-existing occlusion before providing a restoration. Instead it has become customary to provide the restoration and then to 'check' the occlusion afterwards. If this is our habit, we should ask ourselves the question what are we checking the occlusion of our restoration against? It cannot be the pre-existing occlusion if we did not examine it first. The principle of providing a new restoration that does not alter the patient's occlusion is described in restorative dentistry as the 'conformative approach', and the vast majority of restorations are provided following this principle.

The conformative approach

Explanation

The conformative approach is defined as the provision of restorations 'in harmony with the existing jaw relationships'.[13] In practice this means that the occlusion of the new restoration is provided in such a way that the occlusal contacts of the other teeth remain unaltered.[14]

Justification

The answer as to why dentists should wish to adopt this approach is often given as being 'because it is the easiest'. In fact, this is not the

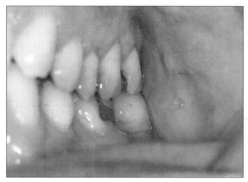

Fig. 1a Teeth touching in CO

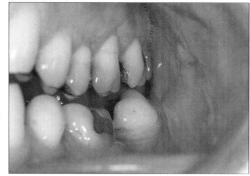

Fig. 1b Premature contact in CR

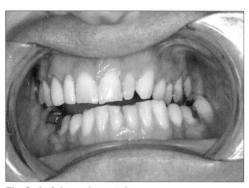

Fig. 2a Left lateral excursion

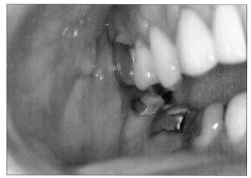

Fig. 2b Non working side interference during left lateral excursion

> ## 'Fingers crossed' dentistry equals stress

> ## Q: When do you use the conformative approach?
>
> ## A: When ever you can

case; the easiest approach is undoubtedly not to consider whether the new restoration changes the patient's occlusion, maybe hoping not to change it too much. The reason why the conformative approach is favoured is not because it is the easiest but because it is the safest. It is less likely to introduce problems for the tooth, the periodontium, the muscles, the temporomandibular joints, the patient and the dentist.

When to use the conformative approach?
The short answer is to use it whenever you can. It is possible to provide a restoration to the conformative approach when:

1. The patient has an ideal occlusion, ie centric occlusion (CO) is in centric relation (CR) with anterior guidance free from posterior interferences. This is unusual, it is much more likely that:
2. The patient does not have an ideal occlusion, but that the removal of the existing occluding surface of the tooth to be restored does not mean an inevitable change in the patient's centric occlusion or anterior guidance. Examples of an occasion where this will not be possible is either if the tooth that is to be restored is a deflecting contact; ie it provides the principal guiding contact from CR to CO, or if the tooth is providing a heavy posterior interference.

    In both of cases shown in Figures 1 and 2 it is attractive to think that all that the dentist has to do is to provide restorations that do

not 'interfere'. The danger in this approach is that the new occlusion may still not be an ideal one, because of the existence of other potential interferences. This new 'less than ideal' occlusion may be a less harmonious one which the patient will tolerate less well ie the possibility of iatrogenic problems may arise.

3. Finally there should not be an existing temporomandibular disorder (TMD). If there is, the decision must be taken whether or not to treat it first, since it is possible that the treatment of the TMD will result in a change of the patient's occlusion.

Improving the occlusion within the restrictions of the conformative approach
Although the principle of not changing the patient's occlusion is paramount within the conformative approach, this, of course, refers to the occlusal contacts that the patient has between their teeth that are not being presently restored. It does not mean that the new restoration should slavishly reproduce the exact occlusion that the tooth in need of restoration has. One of the purposes of restoring it would probably be lost if that was the case. How the occlusion may be improved is best considered within the principles of 'ideal occlusion'.

On the tooth level, ideal occlusion is described as an occlusal contact that is: 'in line with the long axis of the tooth and simultaneous with all other occlusal contacts in the mouth'. This means the elimination of incline contacts. Incline contacts are considered to be potentially harmful, because of the lateral force that they may generate. A lateral force on a tooth may have harmful sequelae, which are illustrated in Figure 3.

So as long as the jaw relationship is the same, it is still the conformative approach. Within the conformative approach it is not only possible, but advisable to improve the occlusion of the restored tooth by the elimination of incline contacts either by careful design of the occlusal platform of the new restoration or by judicial alteration of the opposing tooth.

The acid test is whether or not the occlusal contacts of the other teeth (those which are not involved in the restoration) are changed. If the occlusal relationships of these other teeth are changed then the approach is not the conformative but the reorganised approach. This is not wrong, but requires a different approach and is described later in respect of both simple and complex restorative dentistry.

Technique

Sequence — the EDEC principle

When considering the provision of simple restorative dentistry to the conformative approach, no matter what type of occlusal restoration is being provided the sequence is always the same. The 'EDEC principle' that is presented here (Fig. 4) is a system that the authors have devised to give a logical progression through the sequence of producing a restoration, to the conformative approach. This is capable of modification to other aspects of clinical practice.

The EDEC principle is useful in relation to:

- Direct restorations
- Indirect restorations

The EDEC principle for direct restorations

Examine
Firstly, examine the occlusion before picking up a handpiece. The examination is in two parts: the static and the dynamic occlusions. The examination of the static occlusion in centric occlusion (rather than in centric relation) is done by asking the patient to tap onto thin articulating paper or foil (Fig. 5). Next, ask the patient to slide from side-to-side using thin paper or foil of a different colour; this marks the contacts of the dynamic occlusion .

Design
The clinician must visualise the design of the cavity preparation. This may sound pedantic to some, but it is in effect what every practising dentist does when preparing a tooth for

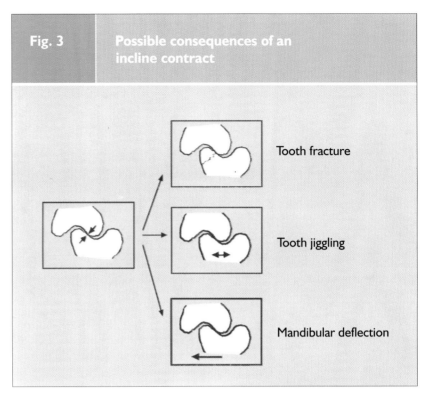

| Fig. 3 | Possible consequences of an incline contract |

Tooth fracture

Tooth jiggling

Mandibular deflection

restoration. The only difference in this sequence is that the suggestion is made that the visualisation is better done after a simple occlusal examination (Fig. 6). The existing occlusal marks will either be preserved by being avoided in the preparation, or they will be involved in the design. As established, they do not have to be exactly duplicated as it may be possible to improve them (from being 'incline contacts' to 'cusp tip to fossa/marginal ridge' relationships), or it may be possible to add an occlusal contact if the restoration being replaced was in infra occlusion.

Often it will be found that the previous restoration is in infra occlusion, as every dentist is anxious to avoid the 'high restoration'. But the avoidance of a supra-occluding restoration by deliberately providing restorations that do not contribute to the overall occlusion is not good occlusal practice.

Execution
The execution of the restoration to the design implies that the dentist will have decided the form of the preparation before starting to cut. It is our belief that this does not take any longer and that it is always easier to work to a plan even in the simplest of restorations.

There will be an overall saving in time, especially if the first two stages are carried out whilst the local anaesthetic is working. The finishing of the restoration is also facilitated if there is a definite aim to the carving or shaping (Fig. 7).

Check
Finally, we check the occlusion of the restoration does not prevent all the other teeth from

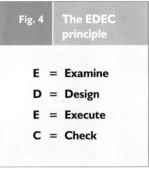

| Fig. 4 | The EDEC principle |

E	=	Examine
D	=	Design
E	=	Execute
C	=	Check

Visualise the end before beginning

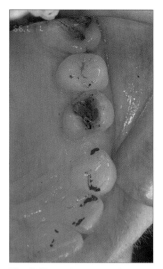

Fig. 5 Shot of pre-existing marks

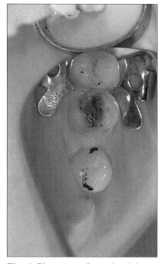

Fig. 6 Close-up of tooth with pre-existing marks

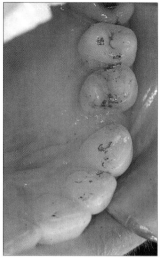

Fig. 8a Initial check of finished restoration

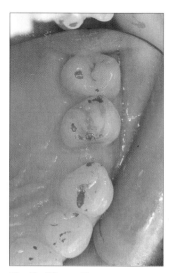

Fig. 8b After adjustment

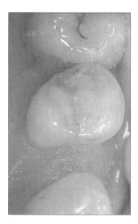

Fig. 7 Close-up of finished restoration

> **There is no point in the technician designing the occlusal aspect of the restoration on models that do not accurately conform to the patient's occlusion**

touching in exactly the same way as they did before. This is either done by referring to some diagrammatic record made, or by reversing the colour of the paper or foils used pre-operatively, or from memory.

In the illustrated case it can be seen that the occlusal contact against the mesial marginal ridge of the restored UL4 (24) is slightly too heavy (Fig. 8a); this has prevented the palatal cusp of this tooth from occluding and has changed the occlusion of the canine. After minimal adjustment, this has been rectified (Fig. 8b). For simplicity of illustration, the dynamic occlusion has not been shown in this series.

The EDEC principle for indirect restorations

The EDEC principle is still followed for indirect restorations (Fig. 9). The essential difference between a direct and an indirect restoration is that a second operator is involved, namely the laboratory technician. We believe that it is a more accurate representation of the working relationship to consider the laboratory technician to be a second operator rather than an assistant, as it makes it clear that the technician also has expectations and responsibilities

Two operators means there are several consequences to the treatment sequence (Fig. 10). The dentist not only has to examine the occlusion but the results of that examination have to be accurately recorded and that record has to be transferred to the technician. This is the clinician's responsibility. Secondly, the technician has the responsibility to preserve the accuracy of that record during the laboratory phase of treatment. Finally, because of the interval in treatment to allow the restoration to be made, the clinician has the responsibility to maintain the patient in the same occlusion during that interval. Consequently it is imperative that the patient is dismissed from the preparation appointment with a temporary restoration which will maintain the same relationship between the prepared tooth and the adjacent and opposing teeth (Fig. 10).

Examine
The examination of the patient's pre-existing occlusion is carried out in exactly the same way as described for the direct restoration. There is a need for that information to be transferred accurately to the laboratory technician: a record must be made.

The provision of an indirect restoration always involves the transfer of anatomical information in the form of the impressions. It is the occlusal relationship of teeth which is the important record, because the technician cannot carry out his or her responsibilities without knowing how the upper and lower models relate to one another.

Fig 9	The EDEC principle for indirect restoration	
E	=	**Examine** and **record** the pre-existing occlusion
D	=	**Design** the restoration
E	=	**Execute** the restoration
C	=	**Check** the occlusion at the fit appointment

There are three ways in which this anatomical information can be transferred: two dimensional bite records, three dimensional bite records, and a combination of both.

Two dimensional bite records

Photographs: It is entirely possible that as instant intra-oral photography becomes more available the clinician will be able to send the technician a photograph of the patient's pre-existing occlusion marked by occlusal registration paper or foil; so that in making the indirect restoration to the conformative approach the technician can see what the patient's pre-existing occlusion was in the mouth (Fig. 11).

Written record: It is quick, simple but effective in some situations for the clinician to simply tell the technician what the occlusion should be when the restoration is finished (Fig. 12).

Occlusal sketching: 'Occlusal sketching' is a technique of recording onto an acetate sheet a sketch of the occlusal marks made in the patient's mouth, by articulating paper or foil, of the static and dynamic occlusion. The acetate strip is designed to be viewed in two different ways: one is appropriate to the clinician treating the supine patient and the other is convenient for the technician to use on the bench in conjunction with the models. The occlusal sketch is an easy way for the clinician and the technician to check that the occlusion of the restoration conforms to the pre-existing occlusion (Fig. 13a–d).

Occlusal sketching is a user-friendly way of recording the patient's occlusion. It facilitates the transfer of anatomical information between the clinician and the technician. In addition, it offers the clinician a convenient way of recording the patient's occlusion as part of the dental records, and this may have medico-legal considerations.

Three dimensional bite records

Bite registration materials: There are many different materials and they all have their pros and cons.[15] Their use is not a guarantee of successful transfer of information; and it is easy to to be fooled that when one material fails to produce a good result that a different material would have succeeded. In reality it is nearly always a misunderstanding of the objective of the exercise that has resulted in an inaccurate record. No particular bite registration material guarantees success.

The objective is to record only the correct spatial relationship of the prepared tooth to its antagonists. Other teeth should contact as before.

The inadequacies of models as anatomical records of the teeth and mucosal surfaces give rise to most of the problems. Impressions often do produce models which are not completely accurate.[16] An incomplete impression of an

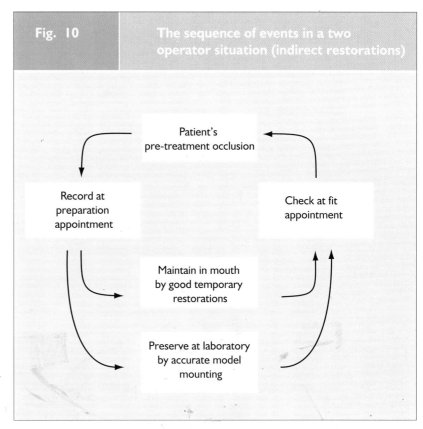

Fig. 10 The sequence of events in a two operator situation (indirect restorations)

Patient's pre-treatment occlusion

Record at preparation appointment

Check at fit appointment

Maintain in mouth by good temporary restorations

Preserve at laboratory by accurate model mounting

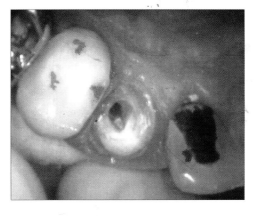

Fig. 11 Intra-oral photograph of occlusal contacts on teeth adjacent to a post crown preparation

occlusal fissure or of an interdental embrasure could very likely result in a significant difference between the occlusion of the patient's teeth and the models. As a consequence the opposing model will not have a true relationship with the working model and it will keep the 'other teeth' apart.

Even if the models are completely accurate and allow the bite registration material to adapt in exactly the same relationship to the models as they had to the teeth, then there is still the problem that in the mouth the mucosal surfaces are soft and compressible, whereas on the models the mucosal surfaces are replicated by hard incompressible material which will probably hold the bite registration material away from its true relationship with the models of the teeth. As a consequence the opposing model will not have a true relationship with the working model: it will keep the 'other teeth' apart.

Fig. 12 — Example of written record of patient pre-existing occlusion

Patient: Mrs Jones   **Job:** crown on tooth LR5 (45)

There are occlusal stops as follows:

Tip of LR3 (43)	against	cingulum of UR3 (13)
Palatal cusp of UR4 (14)	against	distal marginal ridge of LR4 (44)
Palatal cusp of UR6 (16)	against	central fossa of LR6 (46)
Mesio-buccal cusp of LR6 (46)	against	mesial marginal ridge of UR6 (16)

There is canine guidance on the right and left sides

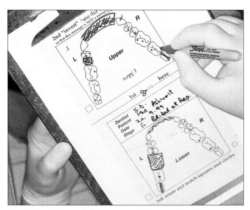

Fig. 13a A sketch is made of the patient's occlusion (before preparation of a bridge) by the dentist at the chairside

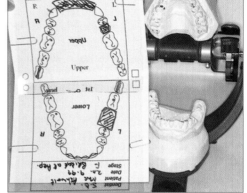

Fig. 13b This sketch is reconfigured at the laboratory as an aid to the technician to confirm the correct mounting of the models

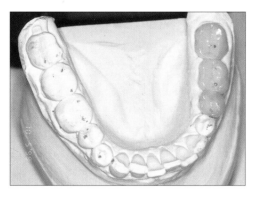

Fig. 13c The bridge is constructed in the laboratory to 'conform' with the occlusion

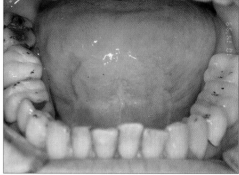

Fig. 13d At the fit stage, the dentist uses the sketch as an aid to check conformity between the pre- and post-operative occlusions

For these reasons, three important guidelines emerge:

- If possible the bite registration material should only be used between the prepared tooth and its antagonists; not used to take a full arch record.

- If a bite registration is going to be used to record the relationship of other teeth it must be carved so that no part of it touches the models of the mucosal surfaces.
- Before the technician starts to use the models to construct the occlusal part of the restoration, the occlusion of those models must be

confirmed against a second record of the bite; and, if necessary, modifications to the models carried out (model grooming).

The 'second record' may be a second bite registration in a different material; for example if an 'easy' material like an elastomer has been used first, it may be wise to use a harder material (in both senses) such as acrylic resin or hard wax. Alternatively the second record may be a two dimensional one, such as occlusal sketching (Figure 13a–d).

The process by which these small corrections are made to the working models or 'model grooming' is discussed under the design stage of the EDEC principle.

Functionally generated pathway

The great advantage of this technique is that it produces a hard record of both the opposing static and dynamic occlusions in only three stages, two of which are carried out in the mouth. There is, therefore, much less room for error. The construction of a functionally generated pathway is often considered to be very difficult and a 'special' procedure in much the same way as the use of a facebow or rubber dam. In reality and in common with these other techniques it becomes, with practice, simple, logical and a time saver.

Technique: A soft, plastic material (eg tacky wax) is applied to the teeth, and the patient is asked to perform a lateral excursive movement on that side. This carves grooves into the wax which represents the movement eg 'pathway' of the lower teeth relative to the upper teeth. This impression is then cast in the mouth using a quick setting plaster applied with a brush. The cast can then be mounted in the laboratory, and used, in conjunction with the 'normal' opposing model.

Alternatively and probably more easily, the patient is asked not only to bite together in centric occlusion (Fig. 14a and b) but also to go into excursive movements (Fig. 14c). A pattern acrylic (eg Duralay)[17] can be built up on a preparation, and then the patient carves out a pathway that the opposing tooth has taken relative to the prepared tooth (Fig. 14d). This record (Fig. 15a) can thus be mounted on to the working model at the laboratory and a cast is produced of the movements of the opposing teeth (Fig. 15b and c).[18]

A functionally generated pathway indicates not only where the cusp tips of the opposing teeth are in centric occlusion (Fig. 15d) but also where they move relative to the proposed crown (Fig. 15e). This is a static record of the patient's dynamic movement.

Dynamic occlusion bite registrations

These are used to anticipate the movements of the opposing teeth during excursive movements of the mandible by enabling the condylar angle to be set in the articulator to the value comparable with the patient's TMJ (Figs 16 and 17).

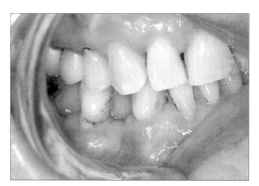

Fig. 14a Patient in centric occlusion

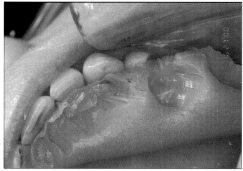

Fig. 14b Wax record of centric occlusion

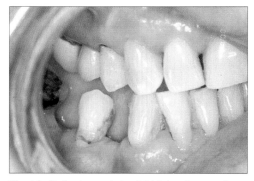

Fig. 14c Patient goes into right lateral excursion

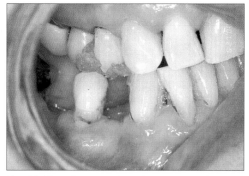

Fig. 14d Duralay recording the pathway of the LR 5 (45) relative to upper premolars during right lateral excursion

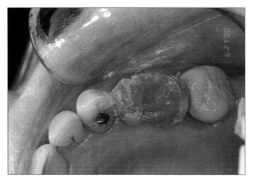

Fig. 15a Set Duralay record of movement of LR5 (45) relative to upper premolars

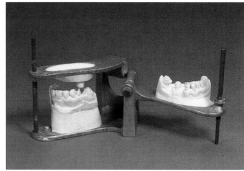

Fig. 15b Twin stage articulator

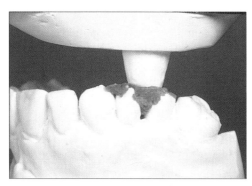

Fig. 15c The Duralay record is used to cast an opposing model

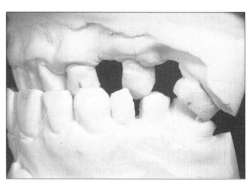

Fig. 15 d Centric occlusion (static occlusion) opposing the inlay preparation of UR4 (14)

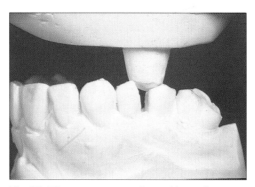

Fig. 15e The movement pathway (dynamic occlusion) of LR5 (45) cast in stone

These records can be avoided, together with their inherent difficulties caused by the compressibility of even the hardest waxes, by either setting the condylar angle to a value that allows some cuspal morphology in the restoration (say 25 degrees) or by setting the condylar angles by simple observation of the space or lack of it between the patient's molars on the non working side (Figure 18a–e).

Design
Clinically the cavity preparation is occlusally designed in exactly the same way as for a direct restoration. The fundamental differences are that firstly the technician is going to make the restoration and secondly that, dependent on the material to be used, there will be certain requirements especially with regard to sufficient clearance between the top of the preparation and the opposing teeth (Fig. 19).

If, because of clinical considerations (eg nearness of the pulp) the clinician suspects that the technician may not have sufficient room, for say an adequate thickness of porcelain in a metal ceramic crown, then it is much better to give the technician permission to reduce the height of the opposing tooth than to risk a high crown. It is essential in this situation, to advise the patient at *the preparation appointment* that adjustment to the opposing tooth may be necessary next time, giving reasons. Alternatively, after discussions between dentist and technician, it may be decided that the best course of action would be to further reduce the height of the preparation. In this circumstance this can be done simply by the use of a coloured separator medium on the die, or very accurately by the use of a transfer coping with an open top made to fit the adjusted height of the preparation (Figs 20a,b).

Model grooming: common sense or heresy?
Model grooming is the title given to the process of adjusting the models so that they more accurately reflect the occlusal contacts that the patient has in their real dentition. Implicit in the use of the word 'grooming' is understanding that these are small not gross adjustments to the occlusal surfaces of the plaster models.

The critics of model grooming have two objections, namely that it should not be necessary and that as soon as the technician or dentist scratches those models, they are not a completely accurate representation of patient's teeth.

Objection No. 1: It should not be necessary.
This objection is quite correct; if the impression, casting and mounted processes have been performed entirely without any error, then the models will exactly duplicate the patient's teeth and the occlusal contacts that the teeth make. Whereas everybody involved in this process of anatomical information transfer should strive for this perfect replication, it is the authors' view that nobody achieves this high goal every time. So it follows that whereas model grooming should not be necessary, model checking is always necessary. This means that, before the models and the relationship between them can be accepted as accurate then some process of verification should be employed (stage 4, Fig. 21). This could even involve recalling the patient, but much more conveniently, some form of second 'check bite' can be used. This may be either two or three dimensional as already described.

If at this verification an error is detected, then the clinician has three choices: do all or part of the process again, engage in model grooming, or proceed with fabrication of the restoration having decided to ignore the error.

Which option is chosen should depend the circumstances of the case; the first and last have definite drawbacks. Which is best depends upon many factors including the size of the error. If the error is gross, repeating the process

may be the only option; it will be inconvenient to the technician, clinician and patient. However, it will take less time than having to remake the restoration.

If the error is small then model grooming is a good option. However, to deliberately ignore the inaccuracy is not a sin; it is simply an admission that the restoration delivered by the laboratory is not going to be as accurate as it could be. Some of the predictability, therefore, has gone, so the expectation of adjustment at the fit stage has increased. In the 'real world', clinicians are constantly having to make compromises; in fact, the skill of a clinician might be judged by their ability to choose and manage compromise.

The clinician who decides to ignore an error at the verification stage, has made a conscious decision to reduce the level of predictable success and is committed to making the adjustments to the occlusal surface of the restoration at the fit stage. The clinician who is ignorant of an error is in uncharted waters and may not even care whether he gets the patient safely into port. It is emphasised that this model verification stage only involves providing the technician with a second occlusal record; this can be a two dimensional record (eg occlusal sketch).

Objection No. 2: If models are 'groomed', then they are not accurate.
This is also true, but if the models are not accurate, the process of grooming is designed to reduce the inaccuracy. As far as the design of the occlusal surfaces of a laboratory-made restora-

> **There is a world of difference between deciding to ignore something and being ignorant of it**

> **Model grooming**
>
> - **Model grooming shouldn't be necessary...**
> - **Model verification is always necessary...**
> - **Model grooming makes sense**

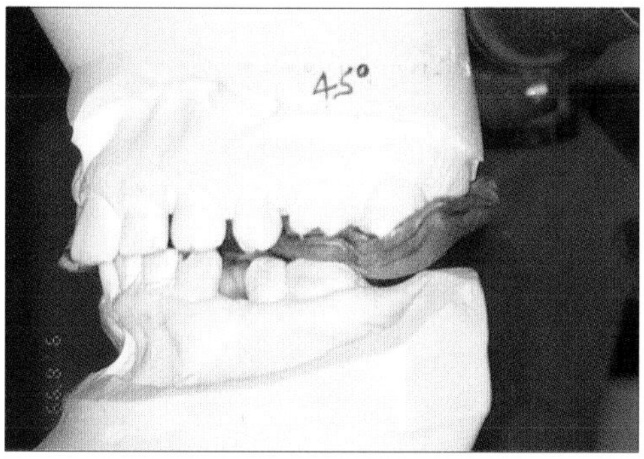

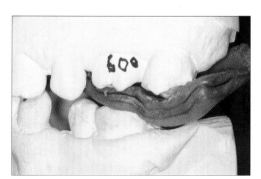

Fig. 16a Wax record is correctly seated...

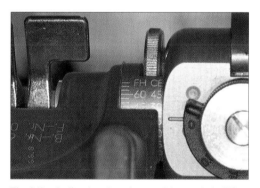

Fig. 16b ...indicating that the condylar angle is 45° (scale FH) Frankfurt Horizontal (KaVo Articulator)

Fig. 17a Wax is incorrectly seated...

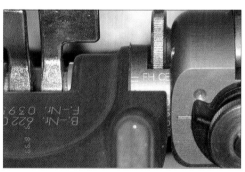

Fig. 17b ...because condylar angle is wrong

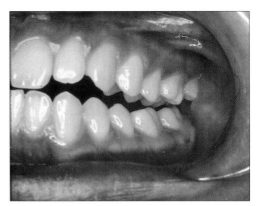

Fig. 18a Gap between patient's back teeth, during a right lateral excursion

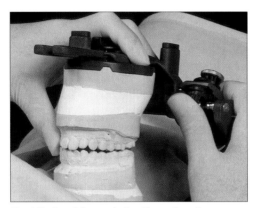

Fig. 18b Condylar angle is adjusted until...

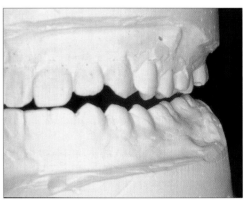

Fig. 18c ...gap on the NWS is the same as in the mouth (see Fig. 18a)

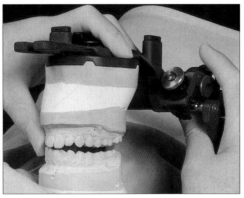

Fig. 18d Too steep a condylar angle...

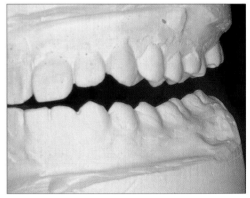

Fig. 18e ...created too big a gap

tion are concerned the only parts of the models that matter are the occlusal surfaces of the other teeth. In fact the only parts that really matter are the occlusal contacts that those teeth make in static and dynamic occlusion. Anybody who doubts this could try the experiment of taking some totally accurate models and drilling holes through the teeth to make them look like Emmental cheese but avoiding the occlusal surfaces. The models would no longer be an accurate three dimensional representation of the patient's teeth but you could still make an accurate restoration on them: only the occlusal surfaces matter.

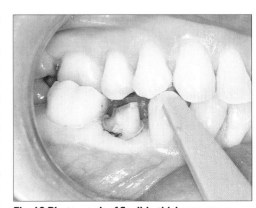

Fig. 19 Photograph of flexible thickness gauge

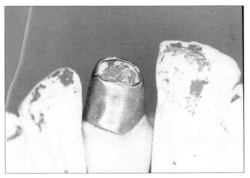

Fig. 20a Transfer coping on die after technician has reduced the height of the core

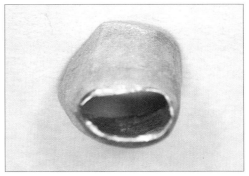

Fig. 20b Transfer coping ready to use in the mouth prior to fit of crown

Fig. 21	The stages before starting laboratory fabrication of the restoration	
1 Impression making	2 Model casting	3 Model mounting
Proceed with laboratory fabrication of restoration	5 Model grooming (if necessary)	4 Technician's verification of occlusion of models against occlusal sketch

Model grooming adjusts the occlusal surfaces of the models so that they make the same contacts as the patient's teeth do. It is part of the '(relevant) anatomy replication' process.

Execute: From an occlusal point of view one of the most significant considerations is the provision of a temporary restoration which duplicates the patient's occlusion and is going to maintain it for the duration of the laboratory phase. For this the temporary restoration should: be a good fit, so that it is not going to move on the tooth; provide the correct occlusion, so that the prepared tooth maintains its relationships; be in the same spatial relationship with adjacent and opposing teeth. By far the easiest way of achieving these aims is to make a custom temporary crown. With a little preparation, custom temporary crowns can be made quite quickly. Figures 22a–d show the preservation of the patient's pre-existing occlusion (Fig. 22a) through the temporisation, laboratory and cementation phases.

Check: The occlusion of the restoration should be as ideal as possible (preferably not on an incline) and should not prevent all the other teeth from touching in exactly the same way as they did before. This needs to be checked before and after cementation. Cementation is the last

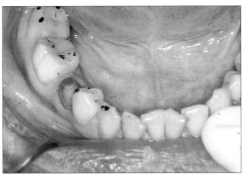

Fig. 22a Prepared tooth with occlusal marks on adjacent teeth

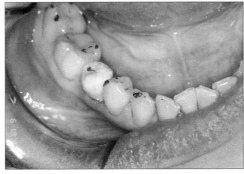

Fig. 22b Temporary crown in place with occlusal marks on adjacent teeth

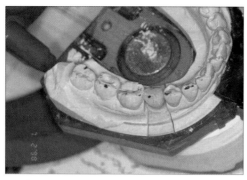

Fig. 22c Final crown on articulator with static occlusion marked

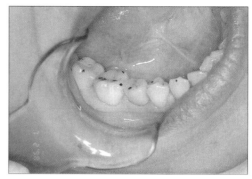

Fig. 22d Final crown in mouth with static occlusion marked

Fig. 23	Ideal occlusion		
Ideal occlusion at tooth level	**Ideal occlusion at system level**	**Ideal occlusion at patient level**	
• Cusp tip to flat fossa contact ie no incline contacts • Occlusal forces directed down long axis of root	• CO in CR • Freedom in CO • No posterior interferences	• Within the adaptive capabilities of the rest of the articulatory system (muscles and TMJ)	

chance we have to get it wrong! If it is a posterior restoration then it is unlikely to be ideal if there is any occlusal contact during lateral or protrusive excursion. Ask the patient to slide their teeth using one colour of articulating paper or foil, and then tap their teeth using a different colour.

The reorganised approach in simple restorative dentistry

The rationale and procedure for restoring a patient to the 'reorganised approach' will be, more appropriately, given in the section: 'Good Occlusal Practice in Advanced Restorative Dentistry'.

In that section, we will be considering the treatment of a patient when the treatment of their dental needs means that it will be impossible to keep the same occlusion and so the jaw

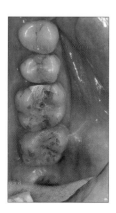

Fig. 24a New restorations are too high

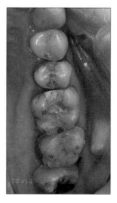

Fig. 24b After adjustment of new restorations, occlusion of adjacent teeth returns

relationship which that occlusion dictates. In that scenario, because inevitably the patient is going to have a different jaw relationship after dental treatment, it is the responsibility of the clinician to ensure that the new occlusion is more, rather than less, ideal in relation to the rest of the articulatory system.

As stated earlier, an occlusal contact that guides the mandible into the jaw relationship is known as a deflecting contact. Some restorative authorities advise that teeth that are not directly involved in the restoration (tooth to be restored and its opposing tooth) can be altered to improve the occlusion, within the 'conformative approach'. We agree that is an attractive idea to try to improve the occlusion of the surrounding teeth, by say removing the incline contacts. The difficulty is to be sure that one is not changing deflecting contacts, because if they are being altered then jaw relationships are being changed. This, then, is not the conformative approach. The objective is now the provision of an ideal occlusion (Fig. 23). For this to be successfully achieved, detailed planning and usually multiple changes in occlusal contacts are needed.

The important limitation of the conformative approach is that none of the teeth to be prepared or adjusted can be deflecting contacts, because if they are then as a consequence of changing them the jaw relationship will probably be changed. If modification to these deflecting contact teeth is envisaged, this then becomes a reorganised approach no matter how few teeth are being restored. This, as will be seen in the next section, is a much more complex procedure.

It can thus be a difficult decision as to 'when to stop' adjustment of the teeth not directly involved in a restoration that is being carried out under the conformative approach.

The new restorations at UL6 and UL7 (26, 27) were being provided within the 'conformative approach'. During the finishing, the occlusal contacts of these restorations are too high (Fig. 24a) because the original contacts on UL4 and UL5 are not evident. After this has been achieved (Fig. 24b), there is an opportu-nity to 'improve' the occlusal contact against the distal part of UL5 (25). This would involve changing it from contacts on the cuspal inclines either side of the marginal ridge to a more 'ideal' single contact on the flat part of the ridge. Although a case could be made for doing so, there is no Figure 24c showing this com-pleted because the clinician decided against it, preferring to leave the occlusal contact at the UL5 (25) exactly as it was before treatment of the teeth distal to it. There would have been a stronger case for adjustment if there had been a single incline contact.

Guidelines of good occlusal practice

1 The examination of the patient involves the teeth, periodontal tissues and articulatory system.

2 There is no such thing as an intrinsically bad occlusal contact, only an intolerable number of times to parafunction on it.

3 The patient's occlusion should be recorded, before any treatment is started.

4 Compare the patient's occlusion against the benchmark of ideal occlusion.

5 A simple, two dimensional means of recording the patient's occlusion before, during and after treatment is an aid to good occlusal practice.

6 **The conformative approach is the safest way of ensuring that the occlusion of a restoration does not have potentially harmful consequences.**

7 **Ensuring that the occlusion conforms (to the patient's pre-treatment state) is a product of examination, design, execution and checking (EDEC)**

1 Beyron H. Optimal occlusion. *Dent Clin Amer* 1969; **13**: 537-554.

2 Celenza F V, Nasedkin J N. *Occlusion. The state of the art.* 1978 Chicago: Quintessence Publishing Co.

3 Dawson P E. *Evaluation, diagnosis, and treatment of occlusal problems.* St Louis: C V Mosby, 1989.

4 Gross M D, Mathews J D. *Occlusion in restorative dentistry.* London: Churchill Livingstone, 1982.

5 Howatt A P, Capp N J, Barrett N V J. *A colour atlas of occlusion and malocclusion.* London: Wolfe Publishing Ltd,1991.

6 Lucia V O. *Modern gnathological concepts.* St Louis: C V Mosby Co, 1961.

7 Mann A W, Pankey L D. Oral rehabilitation. Part 1. Use of the P-M instrument in treatment planning and restoring the lower posterior teeth. *J Prosthet Dent* 1960; **10**: 135-142.

8 Pameijet J H N. *Periodontal and occlusal factors in crowns and bridge prosthetics.* Dental Centre Postgraduate Courses, 1985.

9 Schluger S, Yuodelis T, Page R C. *Periodontal disease — basic phenomena. Clinical management and occlusal and restorative interrelationships.* Philadelphia: Lea and Febiger, 1977, pp 392-400.

10 Schuyler C H. The function and importance of incisal guidance in oral rehabilitation. *J Prosthet Dent* 1963; **13**: 1011-1029.

11 Stewart C E. Good occlusion for natural teeth. *J Prosthet Dent* 1964; **14**: 716-724.

12 Stuart C E, Stallard H. Principles involved in restoring occlusion to natural teeth. *J Prosthet Dent* 1960; **10**: 304-313.

13 Celenza F V, Litvak H. Occlusal management in conservative dentistry. *J Prosthet Dent* 1976; **36**: 164-170.

14 Foster L V. Clinical aspects of occlusion:1. Occlusal terminology and the conformative approach. *Dent Update* 1992; **19**: 345-348.

15 Murray M C, Smith P W, Watts D C, Wilson N F H. Occlusal registration: science or art? *Int Dent J* 1999; **49**: 41-46.

16 Wassell R W, Ibbetson R J. The accuracy of polyvinyl siloxane impressions made with standard and reinforced stock trays. *J Prosthet Dent* 1991; **65**: 748-757.

17 Abadie F R. Plastic stopping — update. *J Prosthet Dent* 1979; **42**: 470-476.

18 Baylis M A, Williams J D. Using the twin-stage occluder with a functionally generated record. *Quint Dent Technol* 1986; **10**: 361-365.

Good occlusal practice in advanced restorative dentistry

S. J. Davies,[1] R. J. M. Gray,[2] and S. A. Whitehead,[3]

In this part, we will discuss:
- The re-organised approach
- When and how to re-organise an occlusion in restorative dentistry

---

In most patients the existing occlusal scheme will be functional, comfortable and cosmetic; and so if a tooth or teeth need to be restored, the most appropriate way to provide the restoration(s) would be to adopt a 'conformative' approach: that is to provide treatment within the existing envelope of static and dynamic occlusal relationships. There will, however, be situations where the conformative approach cannot be adopted, and this section aims to describe what is 'Good Occlusal Practice' in these circumstances.

The 'conformative approach' is not always possible or *appropriate* for 'small cases'

The 're-organised approach' is not always needed or *appropriate* for 'large cases'

[1]*GDP, 73 Buxton Rd, High Lane, Stockport SK6 8DR; P/T Lecturer in Dental Practice, University Dental Hospital of Manchester, Higher Cambridge Street, Manchester M15 6FH
[2]Honorary Fellow, University Dental Hospital of Manchester, Higher Cambridge Street, Manchester M15 6FH
[3]Consultant in Restorative Dentistry, Eden Valley Primary Care Trust, Central Clinic, 50 Victoria Place, Carlisle CA1 1HP
*Correspondence to : Stephen Davies email: stephen.j.davies@man.ac.uk

The term 'the re-organised approach' conjures up ideas of full mouth crown and bridgework even at a differing occlusal vertical dimension. This may be the case for rare situations, but it is not only the 'major' cases that need the extra thought and processes that comprise the re-organised approach. Equally it is often the case that with some care in planning the treatment sequence, apparently complex cases can still be completed within the conformative approach. This will be illustrated in addition to a description of how to 're-organise' an occlusion.

Question: When is the Conformative Approach not appropriate?

1. When it is not possible
This appears to be self evident. However, it is easy to fall into the trap of intending to restore the teeth to the pre-existing occlusion, but to then set about destroying the occlusal surfaces of so many teeth as to make it impossible to return to the pre-existing occlusion when trying to record the inter-arch relationship (bite) later in the treatment sequence.

Changing the occlusion may not be inevitable, even in complex cases
It may be necessary to modify the treatment plan, always leaving sufficient reference points to ensure that as the new restorations are provided they create an occlusion which conforms. For example, preparing alternative teeth at different visits may overcome the problem even in a quadrant in which all the teeth need to be restored. Alternatively, it may be possible to prepare all the teeth at the one visit but safeguard the situation by recording

an intermediate registration after the preparation of only some of the teeth. This intermediate registration then becomes the reference point once the remaining teeth have been prepared (Figs 1 a,b,c).

These approaches are simply examples of following the EDEC principle and may avoid the complication and danger of changing the occlusion, when initially it seemed inevitable.

Question: When is the Conformative Approach not appropriate?

2. When it is not wanted
It may be that the treatment objectives, of the dentist and patient, exclude the 'conformative approach'. Examples would be:

- An increase in vertical height is wanted or indicated
- A tooth or teeth is/are significantly out of position (ie overerupted, tilted or rotated)
- A significant change in appearance is wanted
- There is a history of occlusally related failure or fracture of existing restorations
- Reccurence of a temporomandibular disorder that has relapsed after a period of successful splint therapy.

The vast majority of TMD patients do not need anything other than a period of appropriate splint therapy to provide long-term resolution of their TMD symptoms.[1] There is, therefore, no universal justification for the so called 'second phase of treatment' of TMD involving unnecessary restorations. There will be, on rare occasions however, some patients who maybe need some permanent alteration of their teeth to prevent the reoccurrence of their TMD, and other patients who not only have a

The EDEC principle when restoring complex cases to the conformative approach

E = <u>Examine</u> the pre-existing occlusion

D = <u>Design</u> an operative procedure which allows the conformative approach

E = <u>Execute</u> that plan

C = <u>Check</u> that each stage of the restoration conforms to the occlusion of the previous stage

The reference points of the pre-existing occlusion may be lost with the first sweeps of the air rotor

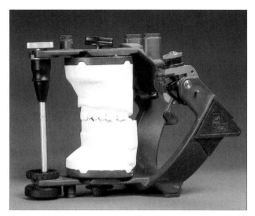

Fig. 1a Pre-operative view before proposed crown preparation of LL4,5,6,7 (34,35,36,37)

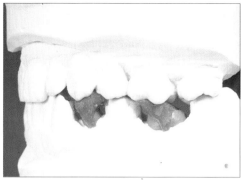

Fig. 1b LL4 (34), LL6 (36) are prepared and Duralay 'bites' taken on these teeth using occlusal contacts on LL5 (35) and LL7 (37) to ensure the 'conformative approach'

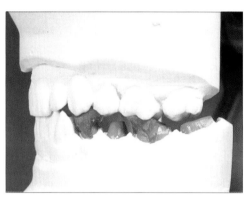

Fig. 1c All teeth are now prepared, but bites against LL4 and 6 ensure models are mounted to pre-operative registration (conformative approach)

primary need for restoration of their teeth but also who have a TMD. These patient, in the authors' opinion, require the closest adherence to the principles of the re-organised approach.

When the Conformative Approach cannot be adopted, there are only two possibilities:

First possibility
Plan to provide new restorations to a different occlusion which is defined *before* the work is started: ie 'to visualise the end before starting': this is *the re-organised approach*.

Second possibility
Change the occlusion, without having planned the new occlusion and the related jaw relationship. To provide an occlusion which does not conform with the previously well tolerated one. This is an occlusion that has been arrived at by accident: ie *the unorganised approach*.

What is the treatment objective of a re-organised occlusion?
At its very simplest, it is to provide restorations, which although changing the occlusion, will be

well tolerated by the patient at every level. No occlusion can be said to be 'intrinsically bad'; an occlusion may only be judged by the patient's reaction to it.

An adverse or poorly tolerated reaction may include the following:

- A temporomandibular disorder
- Occlusal trauma to the periodontal tissues, leading to increased mobility
- Fracture of restorations or of the teeth
- Excessive tooth surface loss
- Hypersensitivity.

Singularly or collectively these represent a most unhappy outcome to dental treatment. The vast majority of dentists who have been actively involved in the provision of extensive restorative treatment plans have some experience of the distress that any or all of these sequalae produces.

For every dentist actively involved in the provision of advanced restorative treatments there is always the danger that a patient will react adversely to our treatment, but we believe that this strategy makes it much less likely. This is because the principle of providing an occlusion to the re-organised approach is to provide an occlusion that is ideal to the patient, *at every level.*

Definition of an 'ideal occlusion', at every level
The definition of 'ideal occlusion' needs to be given at the tooth level, at the system level and at the patient level.

The tooth level
An ideal occlusion will provide:

- Multiple simultaneous contacts
- No cuspal incline contacts
- Occlusal contacts that are in line with the long axis of the tooth
- Smooth and, wherever possible, shallow guidance contacts.

The articulatory system level

An ideal occlusion will provide:

- Centric Occlusion occurring in Centric Relation
- Freedom in Centric Occlusion
- No posterior interferences (anterior guidance at the front of the mouth).

The patient level

An ideal occlusion will be within the neuro-muscular tolerances of that patient at that time in their life. It is only by careful adhesion to the characteristics of an ideal occlusion at the tooth and system levels that one can do more than just 'hope' that a new occlusion falls within the neuromuscular tolerances of the patient.

How to re-organise an occlusion so that it is 'ideal'

Essentially the only difference between the conformative and the re-organised approach is that the re-organised approach is the conformative approach with the extra stages of designing and executing a new occlusion before providing the definitive or 'final' restorations

As soon as these stages have been completed, the emphasis is to ensure that the definitive restorations conform to the design that was planned and executed in the provisional restorations.[2]

The re-organised approach is, therefore, the provision of a more appropriate occlusal scheme prior to delivering the final restoration. It is impossible to confidently proceed directly to final changes in the occlusal scheme and for the most part some form of 'mock up' is employed, usually in the form of a diagnostic wax-up. How to plan and manage the change in occlusal relationships is the challenge. Once the changes are made then the definitive restorations become 'conformative' in approach: that is, conforming to a new occlusal scheme.

It is impossible to make comprehensive *rules* for the management of every clinical situation. However, the following *guidelines* for planning the re-organisation of the occlusion provide a broadly applicable protocol.

Technique

The examination phase

(E = Examine the existing occlusion)

Recording jaw relationships.

The first essential part of the examination is to determine whether the patient's existing centric occlusion occurs in centric relation; if it does not, and assuming that the decision to re-organise the occlusion has been taken, centric relation must be found. The reader will note that the EDEC sequence differs from that in the comformative approach not only in the examination

but also in the execution phase. This is to estimate whether the new (centric) occlusion can be made to this ideal jaw relationship. It is optimal if it can. The difficulty in recording jaw relationships has already been discussed. The use of articulators becomes more critical if any degree of reproducibility is to be achieved in restorative cases where there are major changes to occlusal relationships. The accurate assessment of centric relation may be made more difficult by the length of time that patients have been functioning with their less than ideal occlusion incorporating habitual closure patterns and the guarding of potentially uncomfortable deflective contacts. It is often, therefore, necessary to 'de-programme' the musculature for some period of time before recording centric relation.

Bimanual manipulation of the jaw into a reproducible position can be difficult and some form of appliance may be necessary. At the chairside, an anterior bite plane ('Lucia jig') may be constructed in acrylic resin. This may be worn by the patient for some time in the chair to 'de-programme' the musculature prior to manipulation. Even, this may be ineffective and a stabilisation splint may have to be employed.[3] This is a hard splint made to cover whichever dentition has the most missing teeth and aims to be a facsimile of an ideal occlusion (CO=CR and anterior guidance at the front). It is interesting to consider that the use of splints may comprise part of the examination phase of the re-organised approach, rather than being reserved solely for treatment of a TMD.

The static occlusion is also examined on a tooth level to discover the existence of any incline contacts between the cusps of opposing teeth.

The dynamic occlusion needs to be examined with a view to discovering any posterior interferences on the working (WS) or non-working sides (NWS). In addition an estimate of the condylar angles should be made. This can either be done on a semi-adjustable articulator by the use of latero-protrusive wax records or by simply adjusting the condylar angles of the articulator until the space (or lack of it) between the molars on the NWS is the same as it is in the patient. This can only be done if a face bow record has been used to mount the upper models into the articulator.

The planning phase

(D = design the new occlusion)

It is advisable to accurately duplicate the stone models at the correct centric relation and occlusion on the articulator. A *mock equilibration* can then be carried out on one set, whilst not sacrificing the hard earned accurate record which represents the patient's existing occlusion on the other set (ie the starting point of the treatment). This mock equilibration, involving many small occlusal adjustments, is carried out on the stone models until multiple and ideal contacts

> **'Organise': to give a definite and orderly structure, and to arrange and 'get up' something**
> *OED*

> **'Unorganised': not formed into an orderly whole**
> *OED*

> **The examination phase of the process is completed when the clinician has a set of articulated models that are an accurate representation of the patient's occlusion and jaw relationship**

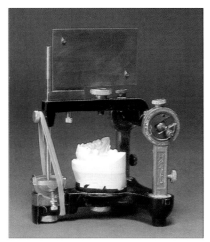

Fig. 2 The flag is attached to the articulator and the incisal pin is set before the upper model is removed

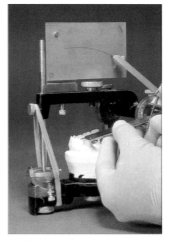

Fig. 3 An arc is drawn on the flag at a set radius using the tip of the lower canine as its centre (Canine Arc)

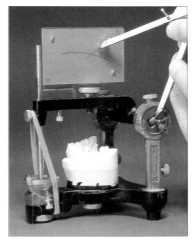

Fig. 4 The canine arc is bisected by an arc using the articulator hinge as its centre. This intersection is the centre of a possible occlusal plane (sphere)

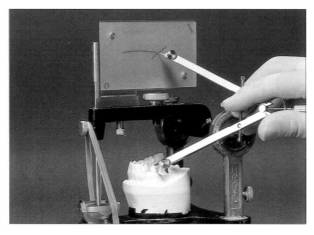

Fig. 5a Proposed occlusal plane obviously still touches the tip of the lower canine

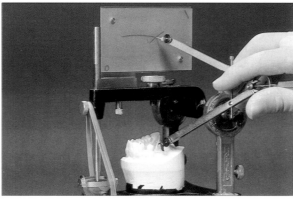

Fig. 5b Relationship of proposed occlusal plane to the mesial abutment and to pontic of the planned bridge

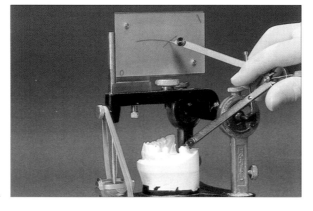

Fig. 5c Relationship of proposed occlusal plane to the distal abutment of the planned bridge

between opposing teeth occur in centric relation. The sequence of these adjustments on the models is recorded as an aid for subsequent clinical equilibration carried out in the mouth.[4]

If the adjustments of the stone teeth exceed that which the clinician judges to be possible or prudent for the real teeth, then an important conclusion will have been reached: that it will not be possible to achieve an ideal occlusion without major alteration to those teeth. This may indicate a need for considering any of the following:

• Provisional restorations of some type
• Orthodontic adjustment
• or even ... extraction.

The next stage in the design of the new occlusion is a *diagnostic wax up*. In this process the correctly mounted and now equilibrated casts are modified by the application of wax as a mock-up of the final restorations or prostheses. It is best if this is carried out by the clinician; but if it is carried out by the technician, the final responsibility of design still rests with the clinician. It is, therefore, of paramount importance that the technician providing the wax up understands that there are limitations to the provision of restorations because it is possible to 'cheat' in the laboratory but not in the mouth. The diagnostic wax up gives positive information on the occlusal scheme that can be generated. It is a valuable guide to the treatment objective for both the clinician and the technician and it should be agreed by both parties before the patient's teeth are touched. The concept of the 'ideal occlusion' should be incorporated wherever possible. The diagnostic wax up can also reveal information regarding the need for crown lengthening and orthodontic tooth movement, in addition to being a wonderful guide to the optimum crown preparation form. A diagnostic wax up will provide the template for the temporary restorations. Finally it gives the patient an opportunity to visualise the treatment and enhance their ability to make informed choices.

The greatest difficulty in designing the occlusion in a diagnostic wax up is to create the occlusal planes. This can be assisted by the use of a 'flag' on the articulator. By the use of this device an approximation of the centre of the curves of Wilson and Spey can be made.

How to use a flag to determine the planes of occlusion in a diagnostic wax up

Step 1. Mount the models on a semi-adjustable articulator, after taking a facebow record and set the incisal pin to record the vertical height, with the models in occlusion. Now remove the upper model and attach the 'flag'. (Fig. 2)

Step 2. Draw an arc on the flag at a set radius from the tip of the lower canine, assuming that the canine is not due to be restored to an increased height. If it is, then a new cuspal tip is waxed up first, and that is used. This is the first stage of trying to find the centre of the sphere which incorporates the ideal occlusal planes. This technique is based upon the long held concept that the occluding surfaces of the upper and lower teeth move relative to each other as if over the surfaces of a sphere with a radius of about four inches, and that the height of the lower canine is the least likely to be changed (Fig. 3)

Step 3. A point along this arc (canine arc) is now found which will be the centre which determines both the antero-posterior occlusal plane (Spey) and the lateral plane (Wilson). As a starting point for establishing the centre of these occlusal planes, the canine arc is firstly bisected by an arc that uses the hinge (TMJ) of the articulator as its centre, using the same radius (Fig. 4).

Step 4. The antero-posterior occlusal plane provided by this centre is tested by reversing the

dividers so the point is placed onto the bisection of the arcs and the graphite end is used to draw onto the lower teeth (Fig. 5 a–c). In this way a harmonious occlusal plane of the proposed restoration can be developed by examining the effect that it would have on the existing lower teeth. At this stage the upper model can be replaced for a similar test, or this examination can be left until the waxing up stage of the treatment planning. The centre of the occlusal planes that is determined by this process is not 'cast in stone', it can be and often must be moved forwards or backwards along the 'canine arc' until an occlusal plane is found that, whilst still an arc, is compatible with the position of the existing teeth. A plane from a centre too far forward will be too traumatic to the opposing teeth (Fig. 6a), whereas if the centre of the occlusal plane was too far back along the 'canine arc' the preparation of the distal abutment would be too radical (Fig. 6b).

Summary

It is emphasised that this technique is suggested as an aid to diagnostic waxing; it is not prescriptive. It does not suggest that occlusions should be restored to a sphere that has a radius of four inches! This would clearly be ridiculous. This technique gives the clinician, who is planning the restoration of an occlusion, the opportunity to provide smooth and harmonious occlusal planes with a predictable effect upon the existing teeth. This information can now be used in the creation of a wax up of the definitive restorations (Steps 5 to 8).

How to do a diagnostic wax up, once the planes of occlusion have been established

Step 5. Firstly cut down the teeth on the lower model, which are destined to be restored, to about 1.5 mm below the proposed occlusal plane. Next add wax to these teeth and any gaps to be restored to a level above the proposed occlusal planes.

Step 6. Use a knife attached to the geometric dividers to trim the wax down to this plane. This will give the position of the cusp tips of the teeth to be restored, on both the curves of Wilson and Spey (Fig. 7a–c).

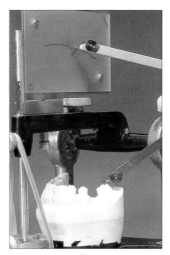

Fig. 6a This occlusal plane would be impossible against the opposing molar

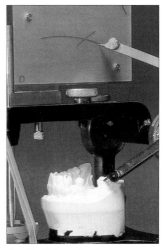

Fig. 6b This occlusal plane would be too traumatic to the distal abutment of the proposed bridge

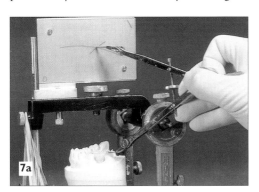

7a

Fig. 7 Wax carved to proposed occlusal planes

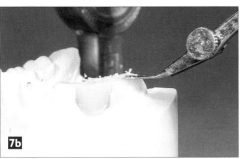

7b

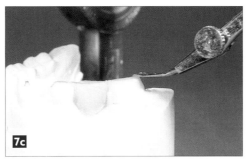

7c

The EDEC principle in the re-organised approach

E = Examine the characteristics of the existing occlusion, including jaw relationship

D = Design and plan the new occlusion

E = Execute the new occlusal prescription prior to definitive restorations

C = Check that you are conforming to this new occlusion in the definitive restorations

Is equilibration possible? Practice on plaster before making irreversible changes in the mouth

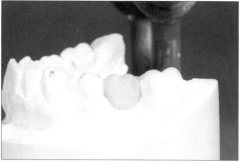

Fig. 8 Morphology is carved into the wax, to represent the final abutments and pontic of the proposed bridge to a planned occlusion

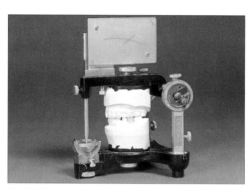

Fig. 9 Minor occlusal adjustment is necessary to the teeth opposing the abutment teeth, whereas the crown on the overupted tooth opposing the gap (in this case) will need to be replaced

Step 7. Carve morphology into the wax to create the waxed up teeth (Fig. 8). (How do you carve an elephant out of a block of marble? Knock off all the bits that don't look like an elephant.) .

Step 8. The wax up of the lower arch is now complete and the upper model is refitted to the articulator (Fig. 9). So that the incisal pin again rests on the incisal table, adjustment will usually be needed to the opposing teeth in the upper arch, this may be minor equilibration or significant change to severely overupted teeth.

Note: These adjustments will need to be made when the lower restoration is fitted; the patient must be advised of this at the planning stage.

Summary

A wax up of a proposed restoration is an ideal opportunity to see the end point of an occlusal change, before picking up a handpiece. The improvement in the occlusion can be developed and visualised (Figs 10a,b and 11a,b)

The pre-definitive restoration treatment phase
(E = executing the planned new occlusion and jaw relationship)

Equilibration (adjusting natural teeth)
Equilibration will already have been performed on the models in the design phase; so the end point and adjustments required to

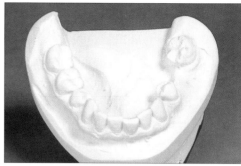

Fig. 10a Pre-operative lower model

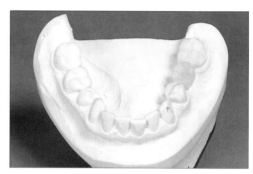

Fig. 10b Lower model after wax up to idealised occlusal planes

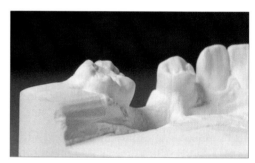

Fig. 11a Pre-operative lower model, illustrating lingual and mesial tilting of distal abutment of proposed bridge

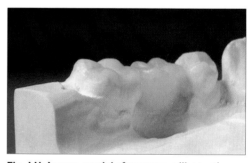

Fig. 11b Lower model after wax up illustrating improved occlusal planes

reach it will already be known. This 'mock equilibration' is highly recommended. It prevents anxiety in the mind of the clinician who when carrying out an equilibration may otherwise wonder whether he or she will be able to finish what they have started! The aim of equilibration is to effect changes in the centric occlusion to give it as far as possible the features of an ideal occlusion:

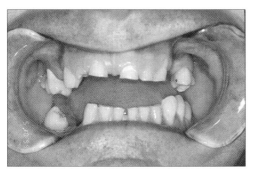

Fig. 12b Patient's dentition exhibiting significant tooth surface loss

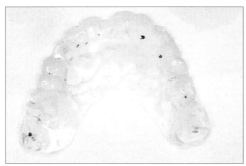

Fig. 12c Upper stabilisation splint with labial veneers to fit over unprepared upper anteriors

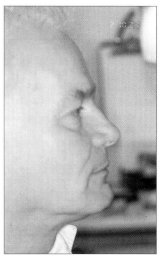

Fig. 12a Patient's profile, suggesting loss of vertical dimension

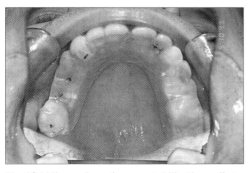

Fig. 12d Mirror view of upper stabilisation splint

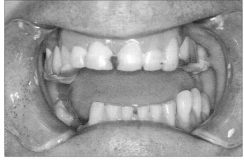

Fig. 12e Anterior view of upper stabilisation splint. Note the provision of median diastema

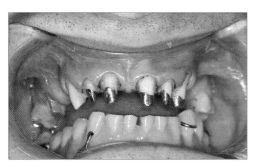

Fig. 12g Definitive lower restoration by partial denture and crown preparations of upper anterior teeth, at the prescibed vertical dimension

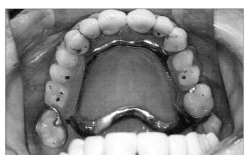

Fig. 12h Mirror view of upper definitive restoration by partial denture and anterior crowns as developed in the 'provisional' phase

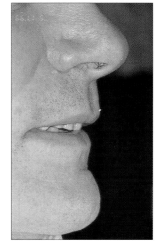

Fig. 12f Provisional restoration vertical dimesion and labial support by the upper stabilisation splint. Compare with Fig. 12a

- Multiple simultaneous contacts
- No cuspal incline contacts
- Occlusal contacts that are in line with the long axis of the tooth
- Smooth and, where possible, shallow guidance contacts
- Centric occlusion occurring in centric relation
- Freedom in centric occlusion
- No posterior interferences.

It may not be possible in every case to provide all of the features of an ideal occlusion. It is inevitable that dentists as restorers and replacers of teeth, sometimes change occlusions. These guidelines are listed to emphasise the point that we should plan to make the changed occlusion as

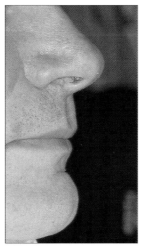

Fig. 12i Restoration of vertical dimension and labial support

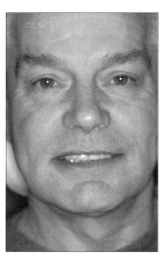

Fig. 12j The re-organised occlusion

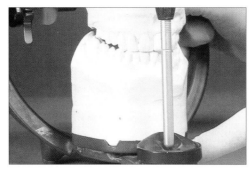

Fig. 13a The models, including provisional crowns on upper anterior teeth, are used to carve a custom incisal guidance table in a slow setting autopolymerising acrylic

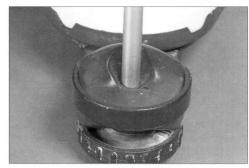

Fig. 13b Custom incisal guidance table. The incisal pin of the articulator is resting in a postion that is related to the centric occlusion of the models

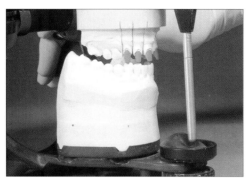

Fig. 13c Custom incisal guidance table is used to guide the upper working model into the same left lateral excursion as was present in the provisional restorations (This would be a right lateral excursion in the patient)

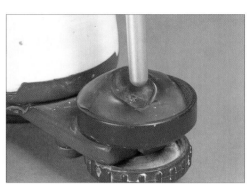

Fig. 13d Close up of custom incisal guidance table, guiding upper model into a left lateral excursion

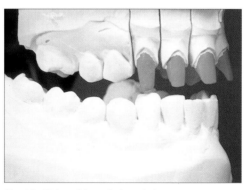

Fig. 13e Using this technique it is easy to see exactly what the crown lengh and palatal contour should be to provide the same canine guidance as was present in the provisionals

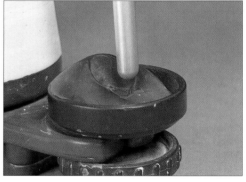

Fig. 13f Custom incisal guidance table determining the lengh of right canine definitive crown

> **The planning and design phase of the process is completed** when the clinician has a set of articulated models and is confident that they are an accurate representation of the end point of the treatment plan

ideal as possible so reducing the risk of precipitating adverse reactions. This aim must be achieved in the pretreatment phase so that the definitive restoration can follow a conformative approach, using the occlusion that has been developed in the design and pre-treatment phases as the starting point.

Simple orthodontic treatment

Teeth may be moved in three planes to a position that is compatible with the aim of the treatment plan.[5] Whether orthodontic movement of teeth is needed is determined at the study model stage.

Provisional restorations

Provisional restorations are always useful and sometimes essential in the management of the re-organised approach. All the information regarding the occlusal scheme of the final restorations should be programmed into the provisional restorations. Subtle changes may be required but the final restorations should conform to the provisionals. The provisions are used to 'develop' the re-organised occlusion.

Cases when the re-organisation of the occlusion includes an increase in vertical height are amongst the most difficult, and so the most essential to plan. The new occlusion including the change in the vertical dimension must be tested (against the tolerances of the patient) by the placing of provisional restorations. A provisional removable prosthesis ie splint,[6] may provide the ideal means of doing this, as it can be modified in the development of the treatment plan. In Fig. 12a–j, a patient with severe tooth surface loss and consequential loss of vertical dimension (Fig. 12a) has been treated initially by the provision of a removable stabilisation splint (Fig. 12c); this was not only the means of testing the tolerance of the new occlusion in three dimensions but also the vehicle to test the anterior aesthetics by means of acrylic labial veneers (Fig. 12d–f).

Once the occlusion has been prescribed in this way, it is relatively straight forward to proceed to the definitive restorations of upper and lower partial dentures and anterior crowns (Fig. 12g–j). In this case, the patient was also able to decide that he preferred not to have the central incisor diastema that had been incorporated into the provisional splint (contrast Fig. 12e and j).

Provisional restorations can be either chairside or laboratory made. Each have their own advantages. Both are adjustable and allow changes to be made until appropriate occlusal contacts and aesthetics are developed. In this context 'appropriate' means 'accepted by the patient.'

The definitive treatment phase
(C =Checking that the definitive restorations conforms to the occlusion that has been designed and executed in the previous phases)

Once the provisional restorations are at the stage when the clinician and the patient are satisfied, they can be replaced by the definitive restorations now using the conformative approach.

It is unwise to proceed with the definitive restorations while the provisional restorations are giving any problems or the patient is not comfortable.

The challenge for the laboratory technician is to 'copy' the occlusal features that have been 'developed' in, and shown to be comfortable by, the provisionals. A customised incisal guidance table is a

good way of copying the guiding surfaces of the upper anterior provisional crowns in order to prescribe the same anterior guidance (Fig. 13a–f).

How to create a custom incisal bite table
A custom incisal bite table is necessary in order to be able to conform to the anterior guidance provided by the upper anterior provisional restorations.

1. Mount models of the completed pre-definitive restorations (provisionals) onto a semi-adjustable articulator, after a face bow record.
2. Lift the incisal pin clear of the incisal guide table by about 2 mm
3. Whilst some autopolymerising acrylic is setting on that table transcribe the tip of the incisal pin through it, whilst guiding the model incisors through excursive movements. (Fig. 13a) This creates a template of the movements of the articulator during lateral and protrusive movement: the custom incisal guidance table is created (Fig. 13b). As the upper models move backwards and sideways (movements which replicate mandibular protrusion and lateral excursion in the patient) the incisal pin of the articulator will move upwards and backwards from the centric occlusion position at the front and bottom of the acrylic guidance template (Fig. 13b).
4. The working model for the definitive upper crowns is now mounted in the same articulator and the custom incisal guidance table is used to guide this model through all excursive movements (Fig. 13c,d). This 'custom' anterior guidance table will now be used to enable the technician to make definitive upper anterior crowns that will guide the patient through the same envelope of mandibular movement as when they had the provisional restorations. It is particularly valuable in setting the ideal crown length and palatal contour of the canine restoration (Fig 13e,f).

Summary
An advanced restorative treatment plan involving the re-organisation of a patient's occlusion

> **The pre-definitive restoration phase of the process is completed** when the patient has an ideal (ie tolerated) occlusion in provisional restorations

> **The definitive restoration phase:** Re-organisation complete — now conform

> **The need for the restorations comes first!**
> - **Ideal occlusion is a concept in the treatment of a patient who needs multiple restorations**
> - **It is not a treatment objective in itself**
> - **A patient should never be provided with multiple restorations solely to provide an ideal occlusion**

A clinical guide to occlusion

1. Davies S J, Gray R J M. The pattern of splint usage in the management of two common temporomandibular disorders. Part III: Long term follow-up in an assessment of splint therapy in the management of disc displacement with reduction and pain dysfunction syndrome. *Br Dent J* 1997; **183**: 279-283.
2. Galindo D, Soltys J L, Graser G N. Long-term reinforced fixed provisional restorations. *J Prosthet Dent* 1998; **79**: 698-701.
3. Howat A P, Capp N J, Barrett N V J. A colour atlas of occlusion and malocclusion. p447-455. Wolfe Publishing Limited, 1991.
4. Parker M W. The significance of occlusion in restorative dentistry. *Dent Clin North Am* 1993; **37**: 341-351
5. Briggs P F, Bishop K, Djemal S. The clinical evolution of the 'Dahl Principle'. *Br Dent J* 1997; **183**: 171-176.
6. Ramfjord SP, Ash MM .Reflections on the Michigan occlusal splint. *J Oral Rehabil* 1994; **21**: 491-500.

is a major challenge for the restorative team. Successful completion will depend upon not only the skill of the clinician and the technician, but also the clinician's planning.

The clinician will need to have:

1. An accurate record of the patient's pre-treatment occlusion
2. A clear idea of the occlusion of the definitive restoration, including the jaw relationship at which it is to occur
3. A detailed sequential plan on how the treatment will progress from 1 to 2, with stated objectives for each phase.

Although it can appear to be a very long way from the starting point to the declared objective, 'every long march has to start with a first step' . If the objective is defined and if the successful completion of each clearly defined step is the foundation for the next phase, success will be the outcome. The key is the sequential treatment plan.

Guidelines of good occlusal practice

1. The examination of the patient involves the teeth, periodontal tissues and articulatory system.
2. There is no such thing as an intrinsically bad occlusal contact, only an intolerable number of times to parafunction on it.
3. The patient's occlusion should be recorded, before any treatment is started.
4. Compare the patient's occlusion against the benchmark of ideal occlusion.
5. A simple, two dimensional means of recording the patient's occlusion before, during and after treatment is an aid to good occlusal practice.
6. The conformative approach is the safest way of ensuring that the occlusion of a restoration does not have potentially harmful consequences.
7. Ensuring that the occlusion conforms (to the patient's pre-treatment state) is a product of examination, design, execution and checking (EDEC)
8. **The 'reorganised approach' involves firstly the establishment of a 'more ideal' occlusion in the patient's pretreatment dentition or provisional restorations; and then adhering to that design using the techniques of the 'conformative approach'**

Good occlusal practice in removable prosthodontics

S. J. Davies,[1] R. J. M. Gray,[2] and J. F. McCord,[3]

The loss of teeth may result in patients experiencing problems of a functional, aesthetic and psychological nature.
This section addresses the very important subject of occlusal considerations for partial and complete dentures. The occlusion is particularly important given the bearing that occlusal factors have, especially on edentulous patients.

In this part, we will discuss:
- **The features of an ideal occlusion in removable prosthodontics**
- **Why these features make it 'ideal' for denture stability**
- **Introduce some techniques for achieving these aims**

Historically complete denture prosthodontics has been at the forefront of the study of occlusion and many of the terms used in occlusion have their origin in this subject. The reason that occlusion has always been a consideration in the provision of removable complete prosthetics is because the adoption of good occlusal practice has a significant and immediate impact on the overall success of the treatment, as it affects denture stability. If an inappropriate occlusion is built into a denture then the patient will be unlikely to be able to accommodate to that denture and the dentist will be immediately aware that the treatment has been unsuccessful. The reason why the correct distribution of occlusal forces is so important in the design of removable prosthetics is because the prosthetic teeth that provide the occlusion *are not directly* attached to the patient.

Students of occlusion have good reason to be grateful to the science of prosthodontics and it remains a part of the undergraduate course where clear guidance on 'good occlusal practice' will be available.

Terminology (see box below)
Terms like 'non-working side' or the more accurate term in a prosthetic sense 'balancing side' are based in a study of occlusion from the perspective of complete dentures and refer to the side of the dentures which are not being used for chewing during a lateral excursion. This can lead to confusion when considering

the temporomandibular joints during that same lateral excursion because the 'non-working side' joint is moving much more than the one on the 'working side'. The terms 'Centric Relation' and 'Centric Occlusion' will be used instead of their synonyms of 'Retruded Contact Position and Intercuspation Position'. Additionally the term 'Static Occlusion' will be used to describe occlusal contacts when the mandible is closed and still, and the term 'Dynamic Occlusion' will be used to describe occlusal contacts when the mandible is moving. These terms will be used in preference to the 'prosthetic' terms of 'occlusion' and 'articulation'.

Classification
Prostheses are often considered under the categories of *partial or complete dentures,* but partial dentures may be supported by teeth, mucosa or a combination of both and, given the fact that the nature of that support dictates the design of the ideal occlusal platform, partial dentures are divided into the following sections:

- Tooth-supported dentures
- Tooth and mucosa-supported dentures
- Mucosa-supported dentures.

Tooth-supported dentures
The concept of the occlusal prescription being 'conformative' or 're-organised' has been discussed previously. The former *conforms* to the constraints of the patient's present occlusal scheme while the latter alters or *re-organises* the current scheme to a more idealised occlu-

[1]*GDP, 73 Buxton Rd, High Lane, Stockport SK6 8DR; P/T Lecturer in Dental Practice, University Dental Hospital of Manchester, Higher Cambridge St., Manchester M15 6FH; [2]Honorary Fellow, University Dental Hospital of Manchester, Higher Cambridge St., Manchester M15 6FH [3]Professor of Restorative Dentistry, Unit of Prosthodontics, University Dental Hospital of Manchester, Higher Cambridge St, Manchester M15 6FH
*Correspondence to : Stephen Davies email: stephen.j.davies@man.ac.uk

Terminology

Centric Relation (CR)	=	Retruded Contact Position (RCP)
Centric Occlusion (CO)	=	Intercuspation Position (ICP)
Balanced Static Occlusion	=	Balanced Occlusion
Balanced Dynamic Occlusion	=	Balanced Articulation

> **In a denture supported by teeth:**
> • **The occlusion is sensed**
> • **The prostheses is less likely to cause instability, if poorly designed**

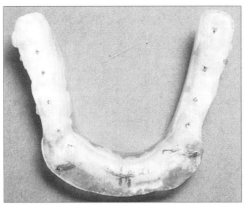

Fig 1 Occlusal diagnostic appliance (stabilisation splint)

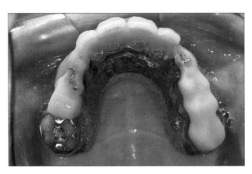

Fig 2 Hybrid prosthesis

sion, sometimes at a raised occlusal vertical dimension. If a partial denture is tooth supported then the design of the occlusion provided by that prosthesis should be to 'conform' with and be complementary to the existing occlusion. The only exceptions to this would be 'rehabilitative' prostheses, which are occlusal diagnostic splints (Fig. 1) and hybrid prostheses (essentially overdentures) (Fig. 2). The difference between the two is that the splint is not intended to be definitive whereas the hybrid prostheses is. Conventional wisdom indicates that the dentist must determine the patient's ability to withstand a raised occlusal vertical dimension with a temporary (diagnostic) prosthesis prior to prescribing the definitive denture/prosthesis.

If a partial denture is totally tooth-supported the patient's occlusion is entirely borne by teeth. This has two important occlusal consequences. Firstly it means that occlusal load will

> **The EDEC principle:**
> **E** = **Examine** the pre-existing condition
> **D** = **Design** the prosthesis
> **E** = **Execute** the prosthesis
> **C** = **Check** the occlusion at completion

be 'sensed' by the proprioceptors of the periodontal membranes. Secondly, it is less likely that a poorly designed occlusion will be immediately manifested by the denture being unstable than would be the case if the support was in part or totally mucosa supported.

Examination
The most important aspect of the examination of the patient, for whom a tooth-borne partial denture is to be made, is to confirm that it will indeed be solely supported by the existing teeth, and not in part by the soft tissues. It is advisable, as in all patients for whom a treatment is envisaged, to carry out a comprehensive examination not only of the dental and periodontal tissues, but also of the articulatory system.

The EDEC principle

E = Examination
The examination of the patient's pre-treatment occlusion is the first stage.

Treatment

D = Design
The support for the partial denture must be provided by the abutment teeth in such a way as to avoid a change in the occlusal contact of the other teeth, otherwise the treatment would not be within the conformative approach. Ideally the rests should also be designed to transfer the occlusal load down the abutment teeth along their long axes.

E = Execute
The design criteria as expressed above may require modification of the abutment teeth and/or the opposing teeth. If this is the case, a clear rationale for the changes can be presented to the patient, and is likely to be much better received than alteration to the dentition after or at the fit of the prosthesis.

C = Check
At the delivery stage, a check is made that the prosthesis has added to the patient's occlusal platform rather than altered its position or dynamic occlusal characteristics. This is easily achieved providing a record of the patient's pre-treatment static and dynamic occlusal contacts has been recorded. It does not matter whether this is a three-dimensional record such as mounted study models on a semi-adjustable articulator, or a two-dimensional record such as a written record or 'occlusal sketch' of articulating paper marks. It is obviously impossible to confirm that the treatment has been provided within the conformative approach unless this pre-treatment record exists.

Tooth and mucosa-supported dentures/prostheses

The mucosa under a denture is capable of displacement to a degree that is 20 times greater than that of teeth via the periodontal membrane.[1] Furthermore there is a difference not only in the amount of displacement under load but also in the type of deformation. The periodontal membrane of teeth, under occlusal force, undergoes a simple elastic deformation whereas mucosa undergoes visco-elastic deformation. This means that the recovery from mucosal deformation is more prolonged than that of a tooth in its socket. These quantitative and qualitative differences between tooth support and mucosa support have an important clinical significance; and obviously could cause problems in the construction of a prosthesis in which the occlusal load is going to be shared between what are two very different tissues.

Examination

The examination of a patient's mouth before the provision of a tooth/mucosa supported removable prosthesis is designed to assess the support, retention and stability provided by the teeth, the ridges and the mucosa. A simple chart is suggested as an aid to this objective (Chart 1).

For a patient with favourable prospects for support, retention and stability of their tooth/ridge/mucosal tissues the chart may appear as in Chart 2. Patient expectations can be better managed if a chart similar to this is used as part of the examination phase

Treatment

The principal consequence of occlusal loading onto the more deformable mucosa will be the loss of occlusal contact. This is a particular problem in patients with free-end saddles. It was for this reason that Applegate described a technique of denture construction,[2] universally known as the 'altered cast technique', which consists of the following stages:

1. Following the recording of the definitive impression, the metal framework is cast and tried-in. If satisfactory, *the saddle area(s) is(are) covered with light-cured denture base material.*
2. The base of the saddle areas is on-laid with light-bodied impression material and an impression recorded of the saddle area *with the dentist pressing on the tooth-borne elements of the framework.*
3. The original master cast is sectioned at the distal abutments and the saddles areas discarded. *The new saddle area(s) are prepared by pouring from this new impression.*

Chart 1 — Simple examination chart to assess potential support, retention and stability before construction of a tooth/mucosa supported denture

	Teeth	Ridge	Mucosa
Support			
Retention			
Stability			

Chart 2 — An example of a completed examination

	Teeth	Ridge	Mucosa
Support	good perio.	square	firm
Retention	good undercuts	favourable	
Stability	good	favourable	

The intention of this technique is to ensure that the occlusal pressure will still be resisted by the ridges after the natural teeth have been minimally displaced into their sockets.

An identical clinical procedure may be undertaken for a reline and this maybe sufficient to restore the occlusion in saddle areas.

Mucosa-supported dentures

Partial dentures

Dentists should be under no illusion that mucosally-supported partial dentures will, within a relatively short time, lose occlusal contact with the opposing arch as the underlying bone is resorbed; this type of denture *cannot* be relied upon to provide a lasting occlusion. In addition, the problem implied in the term 'gum strippers' is well known; a typical example is shown in Figure 3 illustrating the iatrogenic effects of selecting a mucosally-supported design. Simple relines are only likely to *exacerbate* the resorption.

However, not all such designs are necessarily examples of poor dentistry; for instance, train-

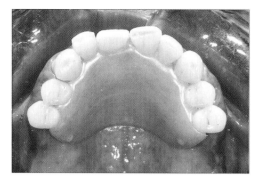

Fig 3 Gum stripper

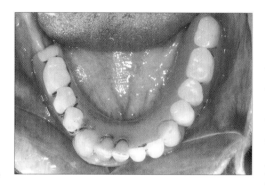

Fig 4 Training denture

ing dentures (Fig. 4) are sensible treatment options when the state of total edentulousness is deemed to be unavoidable.

Examination
It is because of the shortfalls, occlusal and others, that such dentures must only be used *appropriately*. It is, therefore, important that a comprehensive examination of the patient enables an accurate assessment of the prognosis of the patient's dentition.

Treatment
Figures 5 and 6 show an entirely mucosa supported lower partial denture, immediately after having been supplied to the patient (Fig. 5) there is an occlusion between the denture and the patient's maxillary teeth; whereas after 6 months (Fig. 6), there is no occlusal contact against the opposing teeth.

Complete dentures
It has been said that 'a patient with no eyes cannot see, a patient with no legs cannot run, yet a patient with no teeth expects to eat and

act with dentures as with natural teeth'.[3] It is unlikely that this can be achieved, but it remains the goal.

The design of an occlusion in complete dentures is different from that of the dentate patient. While both are concerned with the final act of intermaxillary closure, the absence of direct attachment between the dentures and the patient's musculo-skeletal system requires a different set of guidelines of good occlusal practice.

For all these reasons, it is important to consider the role of occlusion in complete denture philosophy. The fundamental philosophies governing the biomechanics of complete dentures state that there is a fine inter-relationship between support, retention and stability, and the success of the prosthesis will be dependent in a very large part on these features. Importantly occlusion is considered a major factor governing stability.[4]

The *minimal* level of occlusion that any practitioner should prescribe in complete dentures is *balanced occlusion;* this is described by the British Society for the Study of Prosthetic Dentistry[5] as ' even, harmonious bilateral contact between teeth or tooth analogues in retruded contact position (RCP)'. In our terminology this means a 'balanced centric occlusion in centric relation' (CO = CR). This is a 'static occlusion' concept and this type of an occlusion would ensure that, as a patient elevated the mandible into CR, the dentition would be stable. There would be no tilting/displacing force on the dentures and so stability would not be compromised. Factors

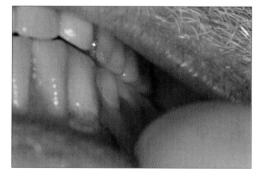

Fig 5 Occlusion at insertion

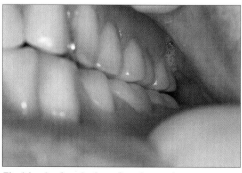

Fig 6 Lack of occlusion after 6 months

For many patients, a simple occlusal prescription is all that will be required, ie the patient has 'evolved' to using essentially vertical mandibular movements with little or no lateral and protrusive mandibular movements.

In this case, no elaborate occlusal scheme is indicated, nor is a semi-adjustable articulator, because the dynamic occlusion can be ignored.

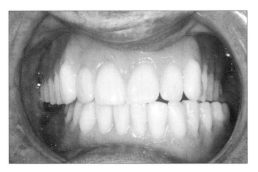

Fig 7a Unilateral prematurity

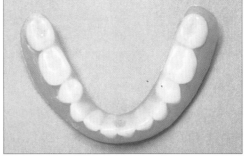

Fig 7b Too large an occlusal table

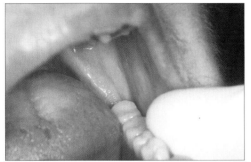

Fig 7c Injudicious placement of teeth

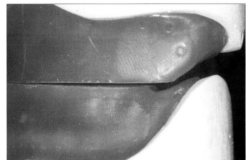

Fig 8 Christensen phenomenon

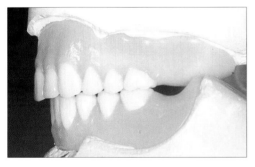

Fig 9a F/F with compensating curves

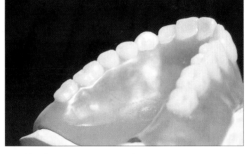

Fig 9b F/F with compensating curves

which might compromise this stability are illustrated in Figure 7. They are:

- Unilateral prematurities
- Occlusal tables which are too large
- Injudicious placement of teeth.

For other patients, however, lateral and protrusive movements are part of their normal 'ruminatory' mandibular pattern and for these patients, a balanced dynamic occlusion *(balanced articulation)* is required. In other words, consideration must be given not only to the static but also to the dynamic occlusal prescription.

In this situation, the teeth of the maxillary denture must maintain harmonious sliding contacts with the teeth of the mandibular denture in all excursive movements otherwise denture stability may be significantly compromised. For example, in a natural dentition, the act of protrusion usually results in a posterior open bite (the Christensen phenomenon — Fig. 8). Such a situation would lead to instability in complete dentures, hence compensating

curves (Fig. 9a and b) are incorporated into the dentures. The same philosophy holds for lateral excursions.

This means that the 'ideal occlusion' for a patient with complete dentures differs from the 'ideal occlusion' for a dentate patient, for example it is 'ideal' for complete denture stability if there is *no* posterior disclusion during lateral excursions, whereas immediate and lasting posterior *disclusion* is usually considered to be ideal for the dentate patient.

It is because teeth on a denture are not attached to the patient's neuro-muscular skeletal system and there is no possibility of neural stimulation via periodontal proprioceptors that the criteria of what makes an 'ideal occlusion' have changed. Although there are mechanoreceptors in the denture bearing oral mucosa, they do not continue to send a stream of impulses to the sensory cortex.

It, therefore, beholds the dentist to determine the occlusal requirements of complete denture wearers prior to prescribing complete dentures.[6] If balanced articulation is required, there is no valid reason for *not*:

- Using a facebow
- Accurately determining condylar angles
- Harmonising the occlusion to match mandibular movements.

Summary
It is a prerequisite, for stability in all complete dentures that posterior occlusal contacts occur simultaneously and bilaterally; furthermore these contacts should occur in centric relation and at the appropriate occlusal vertical dimension. In some patients (those with a ruminatory chewing pattern) it will also be necessary to harmonise the dynamic occlusion in order to ensure denture stability.

Examination of the complete denture patient
The purpose of the examination is to lead to the correct decisions being taken at each stage so that a successful treatment strategy can be made.

The examination of the denture bearing surfaces
An assessment of the denture bearing surfaces will involve assessment of:

- *Shape of the ridges:* Moses suggested a classification of ridge shape and described the retentive and support characteristics of each (Plot 1).[7] The ideal occlusion for the prosthesis will, therefore, relate to the ridge shape.
- *Nature of denture bearing area:* Firm or flabby; and sensitive or comfortable to finger pressure. A sensitive or mobile ridge will require an occlusal prescription that is designed to reduce the transmission of force.
- *Space:* If there is very little space *between* the ridges (usually at the posterior part of the mouth) then the distal extent of the occlusal platform will be necessarily reduced in length. It is better that the dentist discovers this at the examination stage rather than the technician when mounting the models.

The examination of the existing dentures
Do the *existing dentures* exhibit?

- Inadequate freeway space
- Evidence of excessive wear: loss of vertical dimension, crossbite, and anterior posturing

If the answer to any of these questions is 'yes', then the new dentures are not going to be made to the 'conformative approach', but rather the occlusion will be changed ie the ' reorganised approach' will be adopted.

The examination of how the patient masticates
The answer to this essential question will in most cases determine whether the patient needs only a balanced static occlusion in centric relation, ('balanced occlusion'), or whether *in addition* they should have a balanced dynamic occlusion, ('balanced articulation').

In order to determine whether the patient has a chewing pattern that involves essentially only vertical mandibular movements, or also uses lateral and protrusive movements, they must be observed masticating.

This seems self evident, and yet very few patients are treated after determining, by observation, the type of chewing that is used. The appropriate occlusal prescription of the denture cannot be determined without this part of the examination which involves the use of the 'diagnostic biscuit' (Fig. 10).

Treatment
Treatment strategy
This will have evolved during the examination:

Should the conformative or re-organised approach be used?
In the vast majority of patients with a restorative/prosthetic need the *conformative approach* is the method of choice. It offers the dentist the relatively simple task of providing treatment which conforms to the occlusion to which the patient has been accustomed.

In the edentulous patient the *re-organised approach* may be indicated if the patient exhibits:

- A temporomandibular disorder
- A grossly overclosed vertical dimension

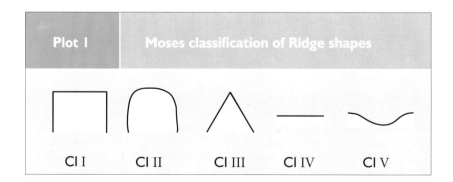

- A pre-existing inappropriate occlusal pattern that has led to denture instability.

If the re-organised approach is to be used; the next question is whether there is a need for a pre-treatment phase of splint therapy. If so, copies of the patient's old dentures will be converted into splints that can be used to establish a new jaw relationship (vertical, horizontal or

> ## The provision of full dentures will involve three stages:
>
> | Colloquial term | Actual function |
> | --- | --- |
> | 1. 'impression making' | designing of the fitting surfaces |
> | 2. 'bite registration' | determining the interarch relationship |
> | 3. 'setting up the teeth' | providing the ideal occlusion |

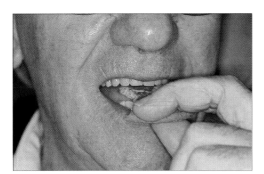

Fig 10 Diagnostic biscuit

anterio-posteriorly).

Does the patient need a balanced dynamic occlusion (balanced articulation), or only a balanced static occlusion (balanced occlusion)?

This question can only be answered by determining, by observation, the type of mastication that the patient employs. This has major consequences for the treatment of the patient, and an assessment, therefore, of the patient chewing is an essential part of the examination of an edentulous patient.

Stages of construction
1. The design of the fitting surfaces
'*impression taking*'
It is the dentist's responsibility to design the denture supporting area on some accurate models and it is outside the scope of this section to expand on this aspect of full denture construction other than to say that it should not be left to the technician.

2. Determining the interarch relationship
'*bite registration*'
The term 'bite registration' is a poor one; as the patient is not asked to bite into anything; in fact if they do, it is likely that they will make an uncontrolled mandibular movement away from CR.

The purpose of this stage is to record the relationship between the upper and lower jaws; in the vertical, horizontal and anterio-posterior planes. Before this stage can be completed, the decision whether to make the dentures to the conformative or re-organised approach must have been taken. In addition, it must have been decided whether only a balanced static occlusion (*balanced occlusion*) or also a balanced

dynamic occlusion (*balanced articulation*) is needed. If balanced articulation is indicated a facebow record must be taken so that the occlusal rims can be mounted into a semi-adjustable articulator.

Gothic arch trace
One means by which a balanced articulation is created on that articulator is the gothic arch trace. This trace is made on a 'central bearing apparatus' (Fig. 11a). This comprises upper and lower acrylic plates onto which is mounted

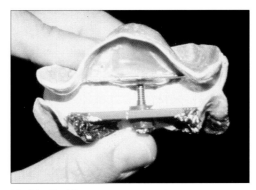

Fig 11a Gothic arc trace apparatus

centrally, a stylus and a platform.

These will record a 'map' of the patient's range of movements, by asking the patient to go into:

- Protrusive
- Right lateral   } excursions.
- Left lateral

The starting point of these movements as inscribed by this trace is the arrowhead (Fig. 11b) and represents centric relation (CR or RCP). If it proves impossible to obtain an arrowhead, this means that the patient does not have a reproducible maxillo-mandibular relationship. This is an important finding and would indicate the need for some further pre-definitive treatment in order to discover a reproducible jaw relationship (ie CR).

This could be achieved by the use of 'pivotal appliances'. A polished pivotal appliance (Fig.12) may look unusual but it is remarkable how well they are tolerated. After fitting, fur-

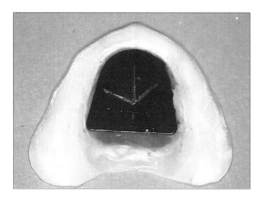

Fig 11b Gothic arc trace arrowhead

ther adjustments are easily made to find the new occlusal vertical dimension (OVD) and to provide occlusal stability. When all adjustments have been made and the patient has been wearing the appliance comfortably for a period, it is a simple procedure to register centric relation with a registration material placed before and behind the pivots. Pivotal appliances may be made on acrylic bases, or from the patient's previous dentures. It may be wise to make a copy of the patient's denture with which to make the pivotal appliance. It will then be possible to return the original denture intact to the patient.

3. Providing the ideal occlusion
'*Setting up the teeth*'

The occlusion of the dentures that will be 'ideal' for the patient is the one which will limit the tilting of the dentures and so minimalise disruption to the peripheral seal, risking instability. As stated this occlusal prescription will take into account the patient's denture bearing tissues and their chewing

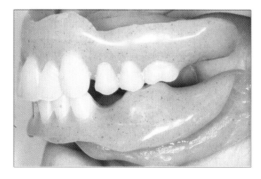

Fig 12 Registering CR with a pivotal appliance

pattern.

On the basis of occlusal form, there are four types of posterior teeth:[8]

- *Anatomic teeth:* these 'duplicate' the anatomical form of natural teeth and typically have 30° to 40° cuspal angles. Modified forms have 20° cuspal angles and these are typically used in complete dentures, on the basis that it is easier to obtain balanced articulation with 20° cuspal angles.
- *Non-anatomic teeth:* these have occlusal surfaces that are not anatomically formed and

are designed with mechanical and not anatomical principles in mind.
- *Zero-degree teeth* and
- *Teeth without cusps:* these may be used for patients who have essentially vertical chewing movements as only their *static* occlusion needs to be balanced (balanced occlusion), ie there is no need for a balanced *dynamic* occlusion (balanced articulation).

In those patients who need a balanced dynamic occlusion, a cuspal form is essential. The dentist has to consider what is appropriate for the patient. If large ridges are present, anatomical teeth will probably suffice. Whereas, if the ridges are flat or where implant-supported dentures oppose maxillary complete dentures, then teeth with non-anatomical cuspal form may be indicated[8,9] as large cusps may induce instability via a tripping effect.

The EDEC principle in complete denture construction (E = Examine, D = Design, E = Execute, C = Check)
The construction of complete dentures is a sequential process. The successful completion of one stage is the prerequisite of starting the next. In order to prevent introducing errors into the sequence it is important to consider what each stage needs to achieve. The EDEC principle is one way of defining the objectives of the process.

E = Examine
The examination of the denture bearing surfaces, the existing dentures and the masticatory pattern will be the basis for
D = the design of the occlusion of the prosthesis.
The first stage of full denture construction is:
E = the execution of that design. This comprises the procedures up to and including the jaw registration. It involves defining the relationship between the denture bearing surfaces in three planes and the design of the ideal static and dynamic occlusion for that patient. At one end of the spectrum this design may be a copy of the patient's previous prosthesis: 'the conformative approach'. Alternatively, there may be need to design changes in the vertical height, jaw relationship and occlusal prescription: 'the re-organised approach'. The design will be achieved and recorded in the jaw registration, when this information is passed to the laboratory technician. From that moment the emphasis of the dentist, during the try-in and completion stages, moves from designing and executing change to
C = checking that there is no deviation from the record supplied to the technician; ie from the bite registration to completion:

'the conformative approach'

Combination syndrome[10]

The final section under the heading of 'mucosa supported dentures' considers the type of occlusion that is required when a full denture is opposed by teeth or a fixed prosthesis, a condition referred as the 'Combination Syndrome'.[10]

There are three scenarios:

1. Complete maxillary denture opposed by dentate/partly dentate mandibular arch.
2. Complete mandibular denture opposed by dentate/partly dentate maxilla
3. Complete maxillary denture opposed by implant retained lower complete denture ('New Combination Syndrome').

Complete maxillary denture opposed by dentate/partly dentate mandibular arch

In this situation, these can be considerable displacing forces on the upper denture resulting from mandibular movements, so the retention of the upper denture must be maximised.

Displacing forces can be reduced by co-ordinating the maxillary teeth and maxillary plane of occlusion to mandibular movement. This is achieved by:

- Using a facebow to transfer the plane of the upper arch to the condylar axis.
- Using a central-bearing screw to create an arrowhead (gothic arch) tracing.
- Setting the articulator condylar angles to accord to the border tracings on the arrowhead tracing.
- Establishing, carefully, at trial insertion, that CR (RCP) is reproducible.
- 'Milling in' the occlusion to suit the patient. This will inevitably be necessary, as cuspal inclines of the denture teeth will be unlikely to be equal to those of the patient's natural mandibular teeth.
- Reviewing of the patient after 3 days to refine the cuspal anatomy.

Complete mandibular denture opposed by dentate/partly dentate maxilla

Success is even more difficult to achieve in this clinical scenario than the former and although similar techniques are recommended, two major problem areas are often present:

- Impaired support potential of the mandibular denture-bearing tissues
- Unfavourable peri-denture anatomical forces, ie muscle attachments.

Complete maxillary denture opposed by implant retained lower complete denture 'New Combination Syndrome'

This third scenario is now encountered with increasing frequency. This application of implants is rightly considered for the patient who is suffering because of their unretentive and uncontrollable lower complete denture. But dentists should be aware of the possibility of the patients developing a 'New Combination Syndrome'.

At its simplest this syndrome will clinically present as ineffective mastication, often associated with a *very unretentive upper denture*. At its most extreme the patient may exhibit periods when they are unable to exert any control over their mandible or find any position where they can rest it, exhibiting a severe mandibular tremor.

The hypothesis on how this syndrome arises is as follows:

As the lower denture becomes more retentive:

- It is *known* that there is a significant increase in displacing forces transmitted to the upper denture by virtue of the increased retention afforded to the lower denture by the mandibular implants. This force may be considerably in excess of the retention that has been provided to the upper denture, a retention that was perfectly acceptable when it was opposed only by a unretentive lower denture on maybe an atrophic ridge.
- It is *thought* that there may be a significant change in the patient's chewing pattern and that this might occur some time after the implant retained lower prosthesis has been fitted.

Before implants were used, the patient probably developed a purely vertical chewing pattern in an attempt to accommodate to the extremely unretentive lower denture. Once the lower denture is retained by the implants, however, the patient may revert back to a masticatory pattern that includes lateral and protrusive movements (the ruminatory pattern of mastication). The occlusion of the dentures, which was acceptable whilst the patient was chewing only with vertical move-

---

Good occlusal practice is different in the edentulous patient from that in the dentate patient.

The form of an ideal occlusion for a particular edentulous patient will depend on their chewing pattern and ridge form

---

Complete denture construction is a sequential process:

- **Examination**   denture bearing surface

    existing dentures

    masticatory pattern

- **Design** the appropriate occlusion

- **Execute** that design

    (up to and including jaw registration)

- **Check** that there is no deviation from that design

    (from registration to completion)

> **As the chewing pattern changes, the features of the ideal occlusal prescription also change**

ments, could now be 'tripping' the upper denture.

Solutions
Some of the solutions include:
- The basic principles of good retention and stability are not only still needed, they are more important.
- The occlusion should be designed to reduce the displacing or 'tripping' forces, even in a patient who appears at the time of examination to have a vertical masticatory pattern ('accommodative chomping').
- The possibility that the patient will need some implants on the upper jaw should be raised, ideally before the implant treatment of the lower jaw is finalised.

Treatment strategies and summary
The principle is to design and provide an occlusion that is *ideal* — ideal for the important criteria of denture success — *stability*. An occlusion is needed that will reduce the displacing forces on the denture(s).

The basic equations are:

$$\text{Force} > \text{Retention} = \text{Instability}$$
$$\text{Force} < \text{Retention} = \text{Stability}$$

The occlusal prescription provided is a major factor in determining the size of the force applied to the dentures. The retentive capacity of the denture is defined by the patient's tissue and masticatory patterns.

> **Force > Retention = Instability**
> **Force < Retention = Stability**

1. Picton D C A, Wills D J. Viscoelastic properties of the periodontal ligament and mucous membrane. *J Prosthet Dent* 1990; **40:** 263-272.
2. Applegate O C. *Essentials of Removable Partial Denture Prosthesis.* pp166-194. Philadelphia: WB Saunders Co, 1954.
3. Applebaum M. Plans of Occlusion. *Dent Clin N Amer* 1984; **28:** 273-276.
4. Jacobson T E, Krol A J A. A contemporary review of the factors involved in complete denture retention, support and stability. *J Prosthet Dent* 1983; **49:** 5-15; 165-172, 306-313.
5. British Society for the Study of Prosthetic Dentistry. *Guidelines in Prosthetic and Implant Dentistry.* pp29-47. London: Quintessence Publishing Co. Ltd, 1996.
6. McCord J F, Grant A A. *A Clinical Guide to Complete Denture Prosthetics.* London: BDJ Books, 2000.
7. Moses C H. Physical considerations in impression making. *J Prosthet Dent* 1953; **3:** 449-463.
8. Lang B R. Complete Denture Occlusion. *Dent Clin N Amer* 1996, **40:** 85-101.
9. Denisen H W, Kalk W, van Wass M A J, van Os J H. Occlusion for maxillary dentures opposing osseointegrated mandibular prostheses. *J Prosthet Dent* 1993; **6:** 446-450.
10. Kelly E. Changes caused by a mandibular partial denture opposing a maxillary complete denture. *J Prosthet Dent* 1972; **27:** 140-150.

Guidelines of good occlusal practice

1. The examination of the patient involves the teeth, periodontal tissues and articulatory system.
2. There is no such thing as an intrinsically bad occlusal contact, only an intolerable number of times to parafunction on it.
3. The patient's occlusion should be recorded, before any treatment is started.
4. Compare the patient's occlusion against the benchmark of ideal occlusion.
5. A simple, two dimensional means of recording the patient's occlusion before, during and after treatment is an aid to good occlusal practice.
6. The conformative approach is the safest way of ensuring that the occlusion of a restoration does not have potentially harmful consequences.
7. Ensuring that the occlusion conforms (to the patient's pre-treatment state) is a product of examination, design, execution and checking (EDEC)
8. The 'reorganised approach' involves firstly the establishment of a 'more ideal' occlusion in the patient's pretreatment teeth or provisional restorations; and then adhering to that design using the techniques of the 'conformative approach'
9. **An 'ideal occlusion' in removable prosthodontics is one which reduced de-stabilising forces to a level that is within the denture's retentive capacity.**

Orthodontics and occlusion

S. J. Davies,[1] R. J. M. Gray,[2] P. J. Sandler,[3] and K. D. O'Brien,[4]

What are the goals of orthodontic treatment?
- **For the Orthodontist**
- **For the Patient**
Are they the same?

*1*GDP, 73 Buxton Rd, High Lane, Stockport SK6 8DR; P/T Lecturer in Dental Practice, University Dental Hospital of Manchester, Higher Cambridge St., Manchester M15 6FH; *2*Honorary Fellow, University Dental Hospital of Manchester, Higher Cambridge St., Manchester M15 6FH; *3*Consultant Orthodontist, Royal Hospital, Calow, Chesterfield S44 5BL; *4*Professor, University Dental Hospital of Manchester, Higher Cambridge St., Manchester M15 6FH
Correspondence to : Stephen Davies email: stephen.j.davies@man.ac.uk

The discipline of orthodontics is directed towards alteration of the occlusion of the teeth and the relationships of the jaws. It is therefore somewhat surprising to find that there is little scientific evidence to support any of the concepts that suggest occlusal goals for orthodontic treatment. Most of the current concepts of orthodontic treatment are based upon personal opinion and retrospective studies. Nevertheless, an attempt is made here to provide a guide to the relationship of orthodontics and the occlusion that is evidence based. Where the evidence is weak, these areas have been highlighted.

The goals of orthodontic treatment for the Orthodontist

The orthodontist's goal of treatment is to achieve as near perfect occlusion as possible. But what is perfection and what is this 'optimal occlusion'? If we examine the early orthodontic literature, we will find that the founder of contemporary orthodontics, Edward Angle, attempted to treat his patients' occlusion with reference to the occlusion of a skull displayed on a shelf in his surgery. This skull was affectionately termed 'Old Glory' (Fig. 1a).

There is no doubt that the introduction of, firstly the six keys philosophy (Fig. 1b), and secondly, the pre-adjusted edgewise appliance designed to achieve them was a quantum leap for orthodontists.

Unfortunately, there is no evidence that achieving this 'optimal' occlusion has any influence upon long-term stability, masticatory function or the alleged association between orthodontic treatment and temporomandibular disorders.

The goals of orthodontic treatment for the Patient

The prime reason for a patient to seek orthodontic treatment is to gain an improvement in appearance. Arguably, we should primarily aim to treat the patient's needs rather than pursue a dogmatic adherence to the six keys of occlusion.

Form follows function

There is fortunately, however, a strong association between the aesthetics of the final treatment (patient's goal — Form) and the achievement of an 'optimal' occlusion (orthodontist's goal — Function). This is because if at least keys 2–5 have been achieved, the patient will have perfectly aligned upper and lower front teeth, irrespective of the relationship between the jaws. In Figure 2, the patient has a 'six key occlusion'. In Figure 3, the patient does not have an optimal buccal interdigitation (keys 1 and 2 missing), yet there is very little perceptible difference in the aesthetics of the dentition.

The need for a full examination

Occlusal examination

It is important to emphasise that it is necessary to carry out a full occlusal examination for all orthodontic patients. It is essential to record

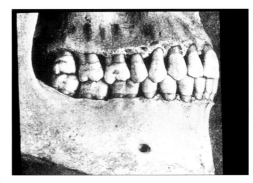

Fig. 1a 'Old Glory': Examination of the dentition reveals that this is, indeed, an 'optimal' occlusion. There is a perfect buccal interdigitation, overjet and overbite. These aims were modified by the concepts of Andrews who introduced the 'six keys of occlusion' (see Fig. 1b)

A clinical guide to occlusion

Fig. 1b	Andrew's six keys to occlusion[4]

I. *Molar relationship:* The distal surface of the disto-buccal cusp of the upper first permanent molar occludes with the mesial surface of the mesio-buccal cusp of the lower second permanent molar.

II. *Crown angulation* (mesio-distal tip): The gingival portion of each crown is distal to the incisal portion and varied with each tooth type.

III. *Crown inclination* (labio-lingual, bucco-lingual): Anterior teeth (incisors) are at a sufficient angulation to prevent overeruption
Upper posterior teeth – lingual tip is constant and similar from 3–5 and increased in the molars
Lower posterior teeth – lingual tip increases progressively from the canines to the molar

IV. *No rotations*

V. *No spaces*

VI. *Flat occlusal planes*

not only the patient's habitual bite (centric occlusion CO or intercuspation position ICP) but also to record the patient's ideal jaw relationship (centric relation = CR or retruded contact position = RCP). This is done against the benchmark of 'ideal occlusion'.[1] Firstly does CO occur in CR? If not, what is the discrepancy between the two? Secondly does the anterior guidance on the front teeth occur with an absence of posterior interferences?

Without doing this the dentist or orthodontist cannot fully assess a malocclusion or avoid a potential mistake in treatment planning.

This is illustrated in Figure 4. In centric occlusion this patient has an overjet of 5 mm and appears to represent a relatively straight

forward orthodontic problem. However, when she is placed into centric relation, the mandible is considerably more posteriorly placed and she has an overjet of 10 mm, which is far more difficult to treat. This is an example of a 'postured bite' and is a relatively common problem in Class II Div i malocclusions. Similar problems may arise from crossbites and premature contacts. As a result, this aspect of an examination is essential if misdiagnosis and incorrect treatment planning is to be minimised.

Examination of the articulatory system

It must be appreciated, however, that the occlusal examination only comprises one part of the articulator system examination; the muscles and temporomandibular joints should also be examined.

The three elements of an examination of the articulator system[2] can easily be incorporated into an orthodontic examination protocol (Fig. 5a–c). This comprehensive examination is divided into two main parts. The jaw and facial examination will record the pattern of the skeletal bases and the facial symmetry, the condition of the TMJs and mandibular muscles, and the soft tissue characteristics. The dental and occlusal examination will record the position of the teeth and their occlusal contacts.

Treatment considerations

Orthodontic treatment methods can be divided into two depending on the goals of treatment,[3] these are camouflage and modification. To introduce this concept we must first consider the aetiology of a malocclusion, which includes skeletal, dento-alveolar and soft tissue components, the first two compo-

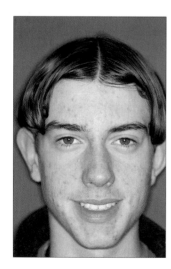

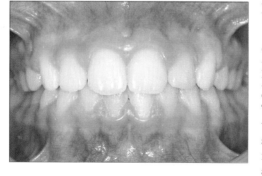

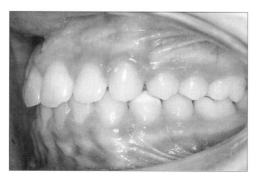

Fig. 2 'Six keys to occlusion' are present (after Andrew); a perfect smile

nents being particularly relevant. An example of the dento-alveolar component is crowding as a result of an adverse tooth-alveolar tissue ratio. When the malocclusion is caused by the skeletal component, the patient typically presents with a discrepancy between the size or position of his or her skeletal bases in the anterio-posterior, lateral or vertical dimension.

At a very simplistic level the orthodontist when faced with these discrepancies has two main choices:

- To provide treatment directed at camouflaging the problem and not changing the skeletal pattern.
  or
- Attempting skeletal modification with either functional appliances or orthognathic surgery

Camouflage
If the treatment is directed at camouflage, space is created in the dental arches by extractions, arch expansion or both, and the other teeth are moved into this space to achieve the treatment objective.

Even if the person has a skeletal discrepancy, the orthodontist may choose to accept the discrepancy and attempt to camouflage the problem by simply moving the teeth.

Unfortunately, whilst the dental appearance can be predicted the facial appearance cannot (Figs 6 and 7). Furthermore, there is no scientific evidence for any technique that may aid in prediction. Some clinicians may say they can accurately predict facial changes, but this claim is totally unfounded.

Modification
An alternative treatment is to attempt to change the skeletal pattern. This may be achieved by 'growth modification' which comprises the use of functional appliances in the growing child pattern (Fig. 8) or by orthognathic surgery, in the adult pattern (Fig. 9).

How does the orthodontist decide on attempting camouflage or growth modification therapy?
There is currently a debate in orthodontics concerned with the detrimental effect of camouflage on the facial profile. Many orthodontists attempt growth modification treatment for children instead. Surprisingly, there is no evidence that functional appliances alter the skeletal pattern of the growing child in any significant way.[5] A recent investigation has shown that most of the change arising from Twin Block treatment is dental tipping with only a small contribution from a change in the jaw relationship.[6] It is still not known if such treatment changes the size and shape of the jaws or purely the relationship of the upper to the

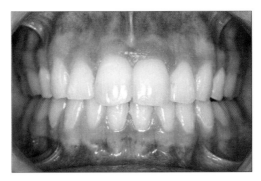

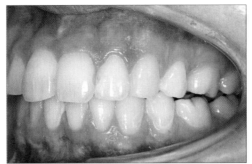

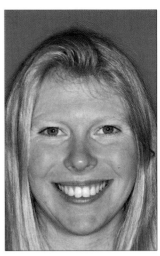

Fig. 3 Not all 'keys to occlusion' have been achieved but aesthetics are still good

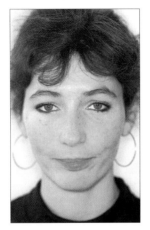

Centric Relation

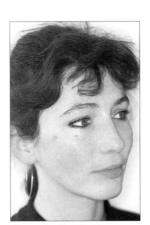

Centric Occlusion

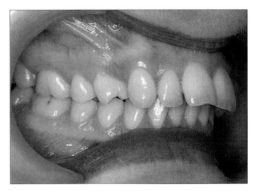

Centric Relation

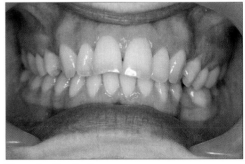

Centric Occlusion

Fig. 4   A patient who has a 5 mm overjet when occluding in centric occlusion and has a 10 mm overjet when in centric relation

> ### *How do functional appliances work?*
> ### Do functional appliances change the position of the teeth within the jaws
> ### *or*
> ### Do they change the relationship between the jaws?

Fig. 5a	Orthodontic examination including articulatory system exam .... Page 1

General Record

Patient   Date

                                              Age

                                    Plaque control   Gingivitis

Medical   good ☐   + ☐
history
                                     mod ☐   ++ ☐

                                     poor ☐   +++ ☐

Jaw and Facial Examination

Skeletal Pattern   I   II   III   mild   mod   severe

TMJ
Tender to palpation?   Lateral pole   Intra-auricularly
                                    ☐   ☐

Noises   Clicks   Right   Left   or Bilateral
                                        Soft or Loud
                                        Consistent or Intermittent
                                        Opening or closing or both
                                        Early   Mid   Late
                                        Painful or Painless
                                        Single or Multiple
                        Crepitus Right Left   or Bilateral
                                        Painful or Painless

Range of Motion (mm)   Vertical maximal ☐   comfortable ☐
            Lateral   Pathway of opening
R ——————+——————— L   straight ☐ or deviating lasting ☐
                                                 or transient to ☐ side

Muscle Tenderness   ## Centre Lines

Temporalis   Masseter   midface ☐

Lateral Pterygoid
                                                 U ☐ ◄—► ☐

Lips Comp ☐   Tongue ☐
                  thrust   L ☐ ◄—► ☐
      Incomp ☐

Fig. 5b	Orthodontic examination including articulatory system exam .... Page 2

Dental and occlusal examination

Erupted teeth

Unerupted teeth

Absent teeth

Upper arch

Crowding   Inclination

mild ☐   none ☐   proclined ☐

mod ☐   spaced ☐   AV ☐

sev ☐ fraenum ☐ retroclined ☐

Lower arch

Crowding   Inclination

mild ☐   none ☐   proclined ☐

mod ☐   spaced ☐   AV ☐

sev ☐ fraenum ☐ retroclined ☐

Incisor Class

I ☐

I/I ☐

II/I ☐

II/II ☐

Overjet in CO

.............mm

If zero
   Freedom in CO?
   Yes ☐ No ☐
Overjet in CR

.............mm

Overbite

Increased ☐

Average ☐

Reduced ☐

Edge to Edge ☐

Complete ☐ ☐ HT

Incomplete ☐ ☐ ST

X-Bites

scissors ☐

displacement no. ☐

.......mm ☐ R ☐ L ☐ ANT ☐

I O T N
   DHC.................
   AC.................

Page 2

If there is a possibility of changing the jaw relationship, the clinician should examine the patient's jaw relationship before and after treatment

61

Fig. 5c	Orthodontic examination including articulatory system exam .... Page 3

Dental and Occlusal Examination cont.

Buccal Segments

Molars

```
        I                    II      III
R     [  ]     .....unit    [  ]    [  ]
L     [  ]     .....unit    [  ]    [  ]
```

Canines

```
        I                    II      III
R     [  ]     .....unit    [  ]    [  ]
L     [  ]     .....unit    [  ]    [  ]
```

Static Occlusion

Does CO occur in CR? ....   IF NOT..prem contact in CR?

Roughly or exactly

Direction of slide from CR to CO ....

Dynamic Occlusion

		RHS	LHS
Non-Working Side Interferences		[ ]	[ ]
Working Side Interferences		[ ]	[ ]
Crossover Position	NWS Int	[ ]	[ ]
	WS Int	[ ]	[ ]
Canine Guidance		[ ]	[ ]
Group Function		[ ]	[ ]

lower jaw. This type of treatment, if it works, does provide excellent dental results (Fig. 8) and, perhaps, reduces the overall time that a child spends wearing fixed appliances.

Orthognathic surgery obviously alters a person's skeletal pattern, however, this is a very complex specialist treatment that should only be carried out, after counselling, for those patients who have major concerns with their facial and dental appearance.

One other form of 'growth modification' is expansion of the dental arches with either removable or fixed appliances. This type of treatment is gaining popularity with many dentists and orthodontists, especially those who attend courses of the latest 'orthodontic guru'.

There is, however, *no evidence* that these appliances can alter the growth of the alveolus and some research has suggested that most expansion is not stable and simply invites relapse in the occlusion.[7]

Extraction vs non-extraction

There has been considerable research into the potential 'harmful' effect of extractions on the dentition, the face and occlusion but it must be emphasised that no scientific study has concluded that orthodontic extractions are detrimental. Unfortunately, the myth still persists and the orthodontists who suggest this type of conventional treatment are frequently described as 'narrow minded' and those who 'do not know any better'.

If a thorough appraisal of the scientific literature is undertaken *no evidence of the deleterious effect of extractions can be found.*

Orthodontics and temporomandibular disorders (TMD)

This link, as always, courts considerable controversy. As discussed there is a tendency to be critical of tooth extraction as part of orthodontic treatment. Implicit in this is the feeling that orthodontic extractions adversely affect the occlusion and furthermore this then leads to a temporomandibular disorder. First premolar extractions are considered by some to be an aetiological factor in TMD, it is suggested that these extractions permit the posterior teeth to move forward resulting in a decrease in the vertical dimension of occlusion.[8]

Another theory is that first premolar extractions lead to over-retraction of the anterior teeth, particularly the maxillary incisors. The anterior teeth then displace the mandible and the condyles posteriorly. Again, it is hypothesised that this may lead to a TMD.[9] These theories may superficially appear plausible. When, however, they are subjected to scientific scrutiny they do not satisfy even the most basic criteria of scientific investigation. The 'evidence' that is commonly quoted is derived purely from personal opinion. Until randomised clinical tri-

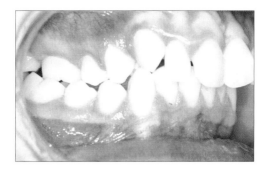
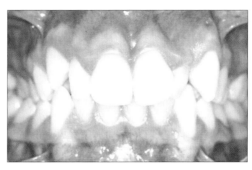
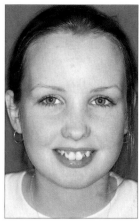
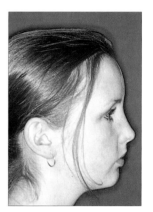

Fig. 6a shows the patient before treament

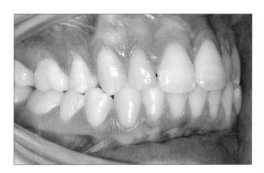
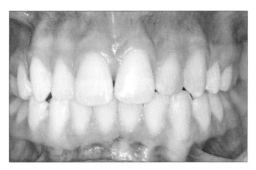
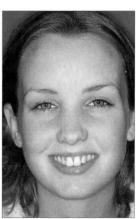
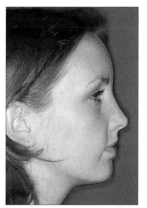

Fig. 6b shows the patient after 'camouflage' treatment. There is a good facial and dental appearance

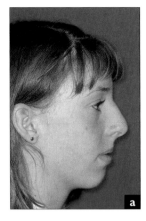

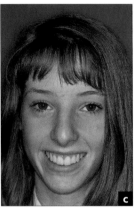

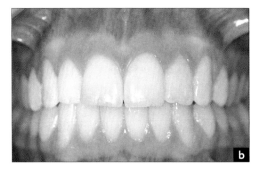

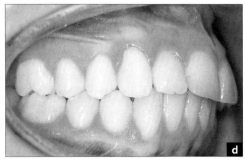

Fig. 7 A Cl 2 div ii following 'camouflage' treatment; showing good occlusion (7b, 7d), but disappointing facial appearance (7a, 7c)

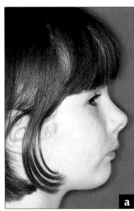

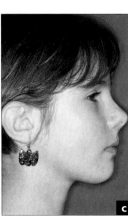

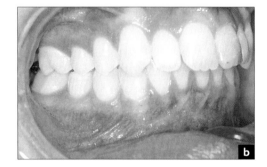

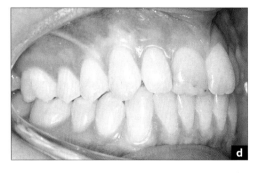

Fig. 8a,b Pre-treatment photographs of a Cl 2 patient before 15 months of twin block therapy; Fig. 8c, d Post operative photographs illustrating good dental and facial appearances

als have been carried out these theories must remain as simply conjecture, anecdotal and lacking in evidence.

Orthodontics and temporomandibular disorders?

Does orthodontic treatment cause TMD?
Clinical experience and review of the literature does not support *any* aetiological relationship.

Can orthodontic treatment cure TMD?
Occasionally orthodontics will form some part of the treatment plan.

Summary

The relationship between orthodontics and occlusion is important. Unfortunately, supposition and hearsay can govern treatment philosophy.

Confining considerations to factors that are supported by scientific evidence, the following conclusions may be accepted:

1. The aims of orthodontic treatment are, surprisingly, unclear. On the one hand an argument can be made for providing a 'perfect or optimal occlusion'. There is little evidence in the literature to suggest that this is necessary. Some features of ideal occlusion do, however, provide optimal aesthetics. This introduces the alternative treatment aim to provide the patient with an appearance that is acceptable to society's aesthetic norms.

2. Acceptable orthodontic treatment goals (including a good occlusion) can be achieved by either the camouflage or skeletal modification approach.

3. Extraction of teeth is needed as a part of many courses of orthodontic treatment. When carried out as a part of a comprehensively planned course of orthodontic treatment, no damage is done to the facial profile or occlusion.

4. There is no evidence in the literature that a treatment plan involving the extraction of teeth is more prone to relapse or predisposes the development of a TMD.

5. An examination of the patient's static occlusion must not only include assessment of the habitual bite or centric occlusion (CO), but also the occlusion in centric relation (CR). This is because the presence of large discrepancies between CO and CR are a positive indication for orthodontic treatment. Equally, such discrepancies should not be introduced during orthodontic treatment. In restorative terminology orthodontic treatment is a 're-organised' treatment plan; and to leave or create a large discrepancy between CO and CR would be to provide the patient with a less than ideal occlusion.

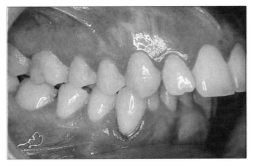
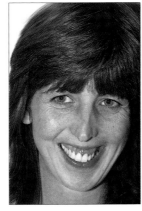
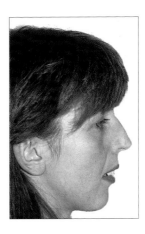

Fig. 9a i –iii Pre-treatment photographs of a Cl 2 patient before orthognathic surgery

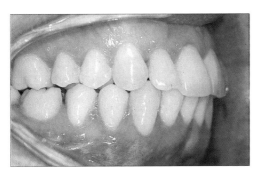
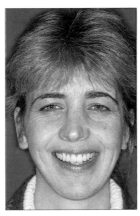
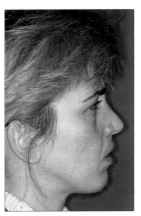

Fig. 9b i –iii Post operative photographs illustrating good dental and facial appearances

Guidelines of good occlusal practice

1 The examination of the patient involves the teeth, periodontal tissues and articulatory system.

2 There is no such thing as an intrinsically bad occlusal contact, only an intolerable number of times to parafunction on it.

3 The patient's occlusion should be recorded, before any treatment is started.

4 Compare the patient's occlusion against the benchmark of ideal occlusion.

5 A simple, two dimensional means of recording the patient's occlusion before, during and after treatment is an aid to good occlusal practice.

6 The conformative approach is the safest way of ensuring that the occlusion of a restoration does not have potentially harmful consequences.

7 Ensuring that the occlusion conforms (to the patient's pre-treatment state) is a product of examination, design, execution and checking (EDEC)

8 The 'reorganised approach' involves firstly the establishment of a 'more ideal' occlusion in the patient's pretreatment teeth or provisional restorations; and then adhering to that design using the techniques of the 'conformative approach'

9. An 'ideal occlusion' in removable prosthodontics is one which reduced de-stabilising forces

10. **The occlusal objective of orthodontic treatment is not clear, but a large discrepancy between centric occlusion and centric relation should not be an outcome of treatment**

11. **An 'orthodontic' examination of the occlusion should include: the dynamic occlusion; and the jaw relationship in which the patient has centric occlusion**

1 Ash M M, Ramfjord S P. Occlusion 4th ed. pp84-85, Philadelphia: Saunders, 1995.

2 Gray R M J, Davies S J, Quayle A A. Temporomandibular disorders: a clinical approach, pp9-25.BDJ publications, 1995, 1997.

3 Proffit W R. Contemporary orthodontics,1st ed. London: Mosby, 1986, p212.

4 Andrew L F. The straight wire appliance. *Br J Orthod* 1979; 6: 125-143.

5 Tulloch J F C, Philips C, Koch G, Proffit W R. The effect of early intervention on skeletal pattern in Class II malocclusion; a randomised contrlled trial. *Am J Orthod* 1997; 111: 391-400.

6 Lund D I and Sandler P J.The effect of twin blocks. A prospective controlled study. *Am J Orthod* 1998; 113: 104-110.

7 DelaCruz A, Sampson P, Little R M, Artun J, Shapiro P A. Long term changes in arch form after orthodontic treatment and retention. *Am J Orthod* 1995; 107: 518-530.

8 Witzig J W, Spahl T J. *The clinical management of basic maxillofacial orthodpaedic appliances.* Littleton, Mass.: PSG Publishing Co Inc, 1987.

9 Fennell M, Frost S. Dentofacial orthopaedics and the GDP Part 3. *Dent Prac* 1993; 31: 8-9.

7 Occlusal considerations in periodontics

S. J. Davies,[1] R. J. M. Gray,[2] G. J. Linden,[3] and J. A. James,[4]

In this part, we will discuss:
- **Whether occlusal trauma is significant in the aetiology of periodontal disease**
- **Whether occlusal treatment is indicated for patients suffering from periodontal disease**
- **Making a diagnosis of trauma from occlusion**
- **Tooth mobility**
- **Occlusal equilibration and the splinting of teeth**

Periodontal disease does not directly affect the occluding surfaces of teeth, consequently some may find a section on periodontics a surprising inclusion. Trauma from the occlusion, however, has been linked with periodontal disease for many years. Karolyi published his pioneering paper, in 1901 'Beobachtungen uber Pyorrhoea alveolaris' (occlusal stress and 'alveolar pyorrhoea').[1] However, despite extensive research over many decades, the role of occlusion in the aetiology and pathogenesis of inflammatory periodontitis is still not completely understood.

Occlusal trauma
Injury to the periodontium resulting from occlusal forces which exceed the reparative capacity of the attachment

---

Periodontitis
The result of an interaction between a susceptible host and bacterial factors in dental plaque, which exceeds the protective mechanisms of the host

---

[1]*GDP, 73 Buxton Rd, High Lane, Stockport SK6 8DR; P/T Lecturer in Dental Practice, University Dental Hospital of Manchester, Higher Cambridge St., Manchester M15 6FH; [2]Honorary Fellow, University Dental Hospital of Manchester, Higher Cambridge St., Manchester M15 6FH [3]Reader in Periodontology, Divsion of Restorative Dentistry, School of Dentistry, Queen's University, Belfast BT12 6BP [4]Lecturer in Oral Pathology and Periodontics, University Dental Hospital of Manchester, Higher Cambridge Street, Manchester M15 6FH
*Correspondence to : Stephen Davies
email: stephen.j.davies@man.ac.uk

Why should trauma from occlusion be considered to have a role in the aetiology of periodontal disease?

Occlusal trauma has been defined as *'injury to the periodontium resulting from occlusal forces which exceed the reparative capacity of the attachment apparatus'*: ie the tissue injury occurs because the periodontium is unable to cope with the increased stresses it experiences. Compare this definition with the one for inflammatory periodontal disease:

'Periodontitis is the result of an interaction between a susceptible host and bacterial factors in dental plaque, which exceeds the inherent protective mechanisms of the host'.

Both processes result in injury to the attachment apparatus because the periodontium is unable to cope with the pathological insult which it experiences. It is quite right, therefore, that dentists should ask themselves two questions:

1. Does occlusal trauma have a role in the aetiology of periodontal disease?
2. Should occlusal treatment be considered for the patient with compromised periodontal attachment?

Before attempting to answer these two questions, the different types of trauma from occlusion need to be defined.

How is trauma from occlusion classified?

Historically trauma from occlusion has been classified as either primary or secondary. *Primary occlusal trauma* results from excessive occlusal force applied to a tooth or to teeth with normal and healthy supporting tissues.

Secondary occlusal trauma refers to changes which occur when normal or abnormal occlusal forces are applied to the attachment apparatus of a tooth or teeth with inadequate or reduced supporting tissues. Recently, the distinction between primary and secondary occlusal trauma has been challenged as meaningless since the changes that occur in the periodontium are similar irrespective of the initial level of periodontal attachment. More usefully, occlusal trauma can also be described as acute or chronic.

Acute trauma from occlusion occurs following an abrupt increase in occlusal load such as occurs as a result of biting unexpectedly on a hard object. *Chronic trauma* from occlusion is more common and has greater clinical significance. In the context of this paper occlusal trauma will mean chronic occlusal trauma.

Question 1
Does occlusal trauma have a role in the aetiology of periodontal disease?
This is a key question because the answer will determine:

- Whether occlusal forces influence the onset of plaque-induced inflammation.
- Whether occlusal forces enhance the rate of periodontal destruction.

Considerable energy has been directed at trying to determine the answer to these questions, because of the possibility that trauma from occlusion *might* contribute to the pathogenesis of periodontal disease. Research studies

A clinical guide to occlusion

designed to examine the effects of occlusion fall into three categories:

· Human cadaver investigations
· Animal studies
· Human clinical studies.

1. Human cadaver investigations
Studies published in the 1960s and 1970s were inconclusive.[2,3]

2. Animal studies
In these studies the variables were the level of periodontal attachment and the characteristics of an applied force, and the way in which it might be varied (See Figure 1 for a summary of the results).

The *periodontal attachment level* is one of three types:

· A normal healthy periodontal support
· A healthy periodontal support but a reduced bone height. This is the experimental model equivalent of a post-periodontal therapy level
· An active plaque-induced periodontitis.

The *type of force* that can be applied to the animal tooth is:

· Either a jiggling force, which is produced by multi-directional displacement of a tooth in alternating buccolingual or mesiodistal directions. This is usually created in the animal by the provision of a supraoccluding onlay.
· Or is an orthodontic force, created by a spring and is a unilateral force that results in the deflection of the tooth away from the force.

3. Human clinical studies
Few clinical studies have identified a clear relationship between trauma from the occlusion and inflammatory periodontitis in humans. A major problem with clinical studies of this type is the lack of a reliable index for measuring the degree of occlusal trauma to which a tooth is subjected.

If trauma from occlusion exists there are obvious difficulties in assessing whether the rate of attachment loss is greater in patients with a continuing plaque induced periodontitis. This is because secondary referral units where the majority of clinically based studies are carried out, do not routinely monitor patients who maintain good plaque control.

On the system level ideal occlusion is or is not ideal for the rest of the articulatory system: the temporomandibular joints and the masticatory muscles. It has, however, been stressed that there is no such thing as an intrinsically bad occlusal contact, because the effect is a product of not only the 'quality' of the contact or contacts but

Fig. 1	Summary of the results from animal studies		
	Healthy periodontium Normal bone height	Healthy periodontium Reduced bone height	Plaque-induced periodontitis
Orthodontic force	Increased mobility Tooth movement No change in position of junctional epithelium or connective tissue attachment	Increased mobility Tooth movement No gingival inflammation No further loss of connective tissue attachment	No progression of periodontal disease
Jiggling force	Increased periodontal ligament space Some loss in crestal bone height and bone volume No loss of attachment Increased tooth mobility which is reversible upon the removal of the force	Increased periodontal ligament space Some loss in height of crestal bone height and bone volume No gingival inflammation No further loss of attachment. Increased tooth mobility which is reversible upon the removal of the force	Gradual widening of the periodontal ligament space Progressive mobility Angular bone loss

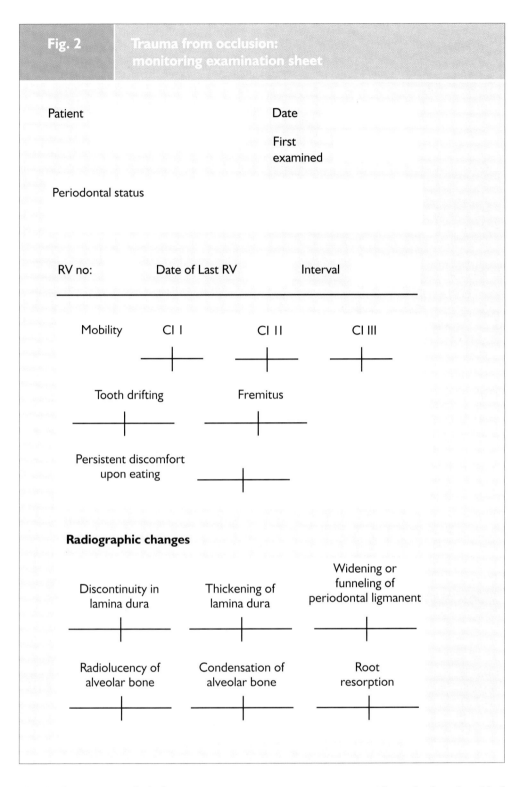

also the frequency at which the contact or contacts are made. Also, it is widely accepted that some patients, at some times will have an articulatory system which is compromised by other factors which reduce their tolerance to a less than ideal occlusion. Factors may range from a systemic disease such as rheumatoid arthritis to the debilitating effects of chronic long term stress.

On the tooth level an occlusion may or may not be ideal for the attachment apparatus, and the same consideration must be given to the frequency of occlusal contact, ie *Does parafunction occur?* In addition, the ability of the attach-

ment apparatus to withstand a less than ideal occlusion may be compromised by periodontal inflammation.

This leads to the second question:

Question 2
Should occlusal treatment be considered for the patient with compromised periodontal attachment?
If it is accepted that increased occlusal forces could result in a further loss of attachment for teeth with an active inflammatory periodontitis, then it follows that a treatment plan aimed

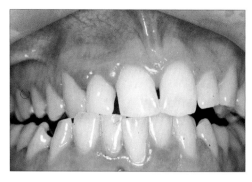

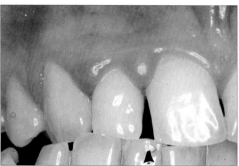

Fig. 3 UR 2 (12) has migrated distally. Examination of the dynamic occlusal contacts of this tooth indicate that the marked wear facet fits closely against those of LR 2 and LR1 (42, 41) during a right lateral excursion of the mandible

It follows, therefore, that even though occlusal trauma is not a proven aetiological factor in periodontal disease dentists as part of their responsibility to help patients keep their teeth for as long as possible in maximum health, comfort and function must carry out a thorough occlusal examination. Treatment aimed at reducing occlusal forces so that they fall within the adaptive capabilities of each patient's dental attachment apparatus will benefit; particularly those with, or at future risk, of periodontitis.

Technique
Examination:
Clinical diagnosis of trauma from occlusion
Increased tooth mobility is not always indicative of trauma from occlusion. It is important, however, that hypermobility which does occur as a result of trauma from occlusion is detected in patients with reduced periodontal attachment. The reason for this is that trauma from occlusion may accelerate further reduction in attachment in a patient with active periodontitis.

A clinical diagnosis of occlusal trauma can only be confirmed where *progressive* mobility can be identified through a series of repeated measurements over an extended period. This means that simple but reliable monitoring needs to be undertaken. A simple monitoring protocol is needed (Fig. 2).

The common *clinical signs* of occlusal trauma are:

- Increasing tooth mobility and migration or drifting (Fig. 3)
- Fremitus
- Persistent discomfort on eating.

The common radiographic signs of occlusal trauma are (Fig. 4):

- Discontinuity and thickening of lamina dura
- Widening of periodontal ligament space ('funnelling or saucerisation')
- Radiolucency and condensation of alveolar bone/or root resorption.

at preserving these teeth must address both problems. This does not mean that trauma from occlusion *causes* periodontitis; rather, it means that occlusal forces may exceed the 'resistance threshold' of a compromised attachment apparatus thereby exacerbating a pre-existing periodontal lesion. While we know that trauma from occlusion can have an effect on the supporting tissues of the teeth, there is no evidence, at present, that trauma from occlusion is an aetiological factor in human periodontal *disease*.

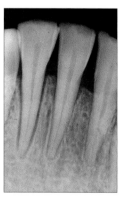
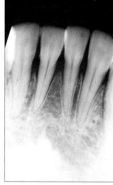

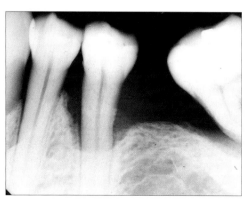

Fig. 4 All radiographs show signs of occlusal trauma to differing degrees

Tooth mobility
Conventional methods for measuring tooth mobility are based on the application of a force to the crown of the tooth to assess the degree of tooth movement in the horizontal and vertical directions. Pathological mobility is defined as horizontal or vertical displacement of the tooth beyond its physiological boundaries. Normal physiological movement is thought to vary between 10 μm and 150 μm and would not be detectable on clinical examination. Clinically detectable mobility indicates some change in the periodontal tissues (ie it is pathological) and the cause of the mobility needs to be diagnosed.

Tooth mobility can be recorded using *Miller's Index:*

I — up to 1 mm of movement in a horizontal direction

II — greater than 1 mm of movement in a horizontal direction

III — excessive horizontal movement and vertical movement.

How can tooth mobility be measured?

Manual evaluation
Manual evaluation of mobility is best carried out clinically using the handles of two instruments to move the teeth buccally and lingually.

Fremitus
Fremitus is the movement of a tooth or teeth subjected to *functional* occlusal forces, this can be assessed by palpating the buccal aspect of several teeth as the patient taps up and down.

Periodontometers
A periodontometer was a research tool used in the 1950s and 1960s to standardise the measurement of even minor tooth displacement. To date, this instrument has been used in a few clinical studies and has limited practical use.

Periotest ®
This device (Fig. 5) was produced in Germany in the late 1980s to provide a more reliable method for determining tooth mobility. It is designed to measure the reaction of the periodontium to a defined percussion, delivered by a tapping instrument. Again this is of limited use in general dental practice.

Tooth drifting or migration
Independent of the state of the supporting tissues of a tooth, if it has moved its position in the mouth, then some force has been responsible for pushing or pulling it. Clearly that force may be extrinsic such as can be seen in pipe smokers or in pencil chewers. Secondarily a soft tissue force may be responsible as with tongue thrusting or lip position (Fig. 6). However, the force may be from an occlusal contact especially parafunction. A frequently encountered scenario is drifting of an upper lateral incisor. This is a common reason for referral of an adult patient to an orthodontist; a referral made usually at the patient's request, with the aim of restoring their appearance. It is important to discover the cause of the drifting before considering any treatment.

Discomfort upon eating
It is important to evaluate how tooth mobility affects the patient. If there is discomfort when

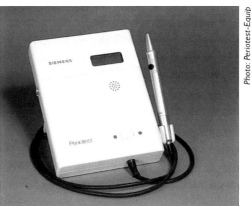

Photo: Periotest-Equip

Fig. 5 The Periotest ® device

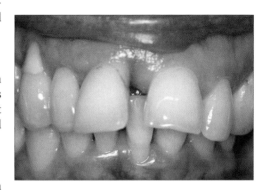

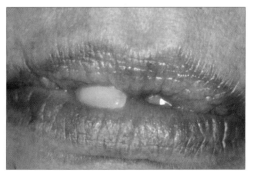

Fig. 6 Initial examination of the UR I (11), in Fig. 6a, may suggest an occlusal cause of the drifting; however, as is shown in figure 6b the reason is the relationship with the lower lip

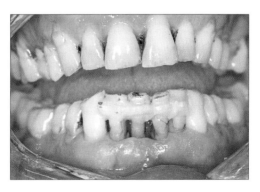

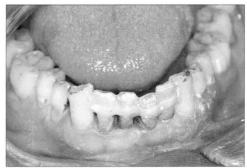

Fig. 7 The lower anteriors have been temporarily immobilised by a labial splint in order to be able to identify the premature contacts and subsequently equilibrate the teeth in order to reduce the trauma from occlusion. (Note: The adjustment to the lower anteriors was only to the labial aspect of the incisal edges: the exposed dentine was already present!)

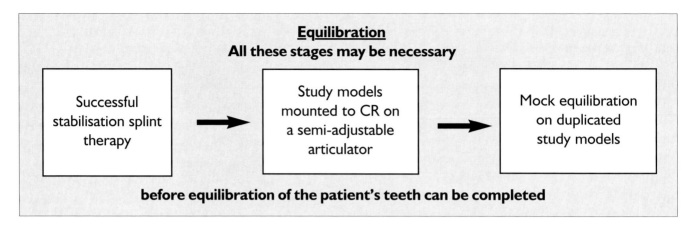

Equilibration
All these stages may be necessary

| Successful stabilisation splint therapy | → | Study models mounted to CR on a semi-adjustable articulator | → | Mock equilibration on duplicated study models |

before equilibration of the patient's teeth can be completed

eating this will have a direct influence upon treatment. The decision will need to be taken, in consultation with the patient, whether to accept the discomfort, extract or splint.

Treatment
(Occlusal considerations in the treatment of periodontitis)

Equilibration
Occlusal equilibration is the modification of the occlusal contacts of teeth to produce a more ideal occlusion.

Is there a need for occlusal equilibration in the periodontally compromised dentition?
The literature does not give an answer to this question. Some studies have shown occlusal therapy to be beneficial in the management of periodontal disease, whilst others have failed to do so.[7–9] Burgett *et al.* reported that occlusal adjustment to reduce tooth mobility *before* conventional periodontal treatment, leads to probing attachment gain after such therapy.[7] The current dental literature, however, suggests that if occlusal adjustment is required it should be carried out *after* periodontal treatment.

There is no evidence at the present time to suggest that occlusal equilibration is an appropriate method for *preventing* the progression of periodontitis. It would, however, be useful to know whether equilibration of a periodontally compromised dentition is beneficial for the long-term preservation and comfort of teeth, in those patients who fail to achieve an excellent level of plaque control.

Equilibrating mobile teeth
In a patient with mobile teeth, it may be necessary to temporarily stabilise those teeth before equilibration is possible (Fig. 7a,b). If a tooth is mobile, it is very difficult if not impossible to effectively modify its shape with the aim of reducing the occlusal forces acting upon it (equilibration).

When to equilibrate (Fig. 8)
Whether occlusal equilibration is indicated will depend upon:

- Whether the inflammatory periodontitis has been treated successfully. If there is an inflammatory periodontal process this should be treated initially. Subsequently when the periodontal condition is stable, occlusal therapy may be necessary for some patients and could involve either occlusal equilibration or splinting.
- The radiographic appearance of the periodontal support. Occlusal equilibration is considered an effective form of therapy for teeth with increased mobility which has developed together with an *increase in the width* of the periodontal ligament (PDL). Reducing the occlusal interference on a tooth with normal bone support will normalise the width and height of the PDL. Eliminating any occlusal interferences for a tooth which has a reduced bone height as a result of periodontal disease will result in bone formation and remodelling of the alveolus only to the pre-trauma level.

  In contrast, if the hypermobile tooth has reduced bone height *but normal periodontal ligament width,* then elimination of occlusal trauma will not alter the mobility of the tooth. In this situation occlusal equilibration is only indicated if the patient is complaining of loss of function or discomfort.

Occlusal therapy in a periodontal treatment plan is established practice
'The World Workshop of the American Academy of Periodontology',[13] issued some guidelines for situations when occlusal equilibration may be indicated:

- When there are occlusal contact relationships that cause trauma to the periodontium, joints, muscles or soft tissues
- When there are interferences that aggravate parafunction
- As an aid to splint therapy.

Splinting
When should teeth be splinted together in the patient with reduced periodontal support? (Fig. 8)

Also outlined[13] were some indications for

Fig. 8	Indications for occlusal treatment and splinting[4,8–11]		
Clinical features	*Radiographic features*	*Treatment required in addition to periodontal therapy*	*Treatment outcome*
Increased mobility	Increased width of PDL Normal bone height	Occlusal equilibration	Normalises PDL width.
Increased mobility	Increased width of PDL Reduced bone height	Occlusal equilibration	Bone fill of angular defect. Bone level stabilised. Normal width PDL
Increased mobility Patient NOT functioning comfortably	Normal width of PDL Reduced bone height	Occlusal equilibration ± splinting	Patient's comfort and function may improve. (This is not periodontal therapy, but an adjunct to it)
Increased mobility Patient functioning comfortably	Normal width of PDL Reduced bone height	No occlusal adjustment required	No further deterioration

splinting, not only restricted to patients with reduced periodontal support:

- To stabilise teeth with increased mobility that have not responded to occlusal adjustment and periodontal treatment
- To prevent tipping or drifting of teeth and the overeruption of unopposed teeth
- To stabilise teeth after orthodontic treatment
- To stabilise teeth following acute trauma.

The first guideline refers to patients with reduced periodontal support. There are two situations in which splinting may be beneficial:

- Where tooth mobility is progressive with increased periodontal ligament width and reduced bone height then splinting is indicated as part of periodontal therapy.
- When patient comfort and function will be improved by splinting, then it is indicated, as an adjunct to periodontal therapy.

This means that if periodontal treatment results in a stable periodontal condition which is comfortable, splinting is not needed.

Summary: Trauma from occlusion in the aetiology and treatment of periodontal disease

- There is no scientific evidence to show that trauma from occlusion causes gingivitis or periodontitis or accelerates the progression of gingivitis to periodontitis.
- The periodontal ligament physiologically adapts to increased occlusal loading by resorption of the alveolar crestal bone resulting in increased tooth mobility. This is *occlusal trauma* and is reversible if the occlusal force is reduced.
- Occlusal trauma may be a co-factor which can increase the rate of progression of an existing periodontal disease.
- There is a place for occlusal therapy in the management of periodontitis, especially when related to the patient's comfort and function.
- Occlusal therapy is not a substitute for conventional methods of resolving plaque-induced inflammation.

1 Karolyi M. Beobachtungen uber Pyorrhoea alveolaris. *Ost-Unt Vjschr Zahnheilk* 1901; **17**: 279.

2 Glickman I, Smulow J B. Alteration in the pathway of gingival inflammation into the underlying tissues induced by excessive occlusal forces. *J Periodontol* 1962; **33**: 8-13.

3 Waerhaug J. The infrabony pocket and its relationship to trauma from occlusion and subgingival plaque. *J Periodontol* 1979; **50**: 355-365.

4 Green M S, Levine D F. Occlusion and the periodontium: A review and rationale for treatment. *J Calif Dent Assoc* 1996; **24**: 19-27.

5 Jin L J, Cao C F. Clinical diagnosis of trauma from occlusion and its relation with severity of periodontitis. *J Clin Perio* 1992; **19**: 92-97.

6 Philstrom B L, Anderson K A, Aeppli D, Shafter E M. Association between signs of trauma from occlusion and periodontitis. *J Periodontol* 1986; **57**: 1-6.

7 Burgett F G, Ramford S T, Nissle R R, Morrison E C, Charbeneau T D, Caffesse R G. A randomised trial of occlusal adjustment in the treatment of periodontitis patients. *J Clin Periodontol* 1992; **19**: 381-388.

8 Galler C, Selipsky H, Philips C, Amnons W F Jr. The effects of splinting on tooth mobility. II. After osseous surgery. *J Clin Periodontol* 1979; **6**: 317-333.

9 Linde J, Nyman S. *Clinical Periodontology and Implant Dentistry.* 3rd Ed. Ch 23: Occlusal Therapy pp711-726 Copenhagen: Munksgaard, 1997.

10 Svanberg G K, King G T, Gibbs C H. Occlusal considerations in periodontology. *Periodontol 2000* 1995; **9**: 106-117.

11 Walton G, Heasman P. The role of occlusion in periodontal disease. *Dent Update* 1998; **25**: 209-216.

12 Polson A M, Zander H A. The effect of periodontal trauma upon infrabony pockets. *J Periodontol* 1983; **54**: 586-592.

13 *Proceedings of the World Workshop in Clinical Periodontics.* Chicago. Consensus report: Occlusal Trauma. The American Academy of Periodontology 1989: III-1/III-23.

Guidelines of good occlusal practice

1 The examination of the patient involves the teeth, periodontal tissues and articulatory system.

2 There is no such thing as an intrinsically bad occlusal contact, only an intolerable number of times to parafunction on it.

3 The patient's occlusion should be recorded, before any treatment is started.

4 Compare the patient's occlusion against the benchmark of ideal occlusion.

5 A simple, two dimensional means of recording the patient's occlusion before, during and after treatment is an aid to good occlusal practice.

6 The conformative approach is the safest way of ensuring that the occlusion of a restoration does not have potentially harmful consequences.

7 Ensuring that the occlusion conforms (to the patient's pre-treatment state) is a product of examination, design, execution and checking (EDEC)

8 The 'reorganised approach' involves firstly the establishment of a 'more ideal' occlusion in the patient's pretreatment teeth or provisional restorations; and then adhering to that design using the techniques of the 'conformative approach'

9. An 'ideal occlusion' in removable prosthodontics is one which reduced de-stabilising forces

10. The occlusal objective of orthodontic treatment is not clear, but a large discrepancy between centric occlusion and centric relation should not be an outcome of treatment

11.   An 'orthodontic' examination of the occlusion should include: the dynamic occlusion; and the jaw relationship in which the patient has centric occlusion

12. **The occlusion of periodontally compromised teeth should be designed to reduce the forces to be within the adaptive capabilities of the damaged periodontia**

Good occlusal practice in children's dentistry

S. J. Davies,[1] R. J. M. Gray,[2] and I. C. Mackie,[3]

The difference between paediatric dentistry and most other branches of dentistry is that in the child the occlusion is changing. Consequently 'Good Occlusal Practice' in children is a matter of making the right clinical decisions for the *future occlusion*. The clinician needs to be able to predict the influence that different treatment options will have on the occlusion when the child's development is complete.

In this part, we will discuss:
- **Why occlusal considerations are different in children**
- **How the adult occlusion can be influenced by the treatment of common problems in the child's dentition**

[1*]GDP, 73 Buxton Rd, High Lane, Stockport SK6 8DR; P/T Lecturer in Dental Practice, University Dental Hospital of Manchester, Higher Cambridge St., Manchester M15 6FH; [2]Honorary Fellow, University Dental Hospital of Manchester, Higher Cambridge St., Manchester M15 6FH [3]Senior Lecturer/Honorary Consultant, Unit of Paediatric Dentistry, Department of Dental Medicine and Surgery, University Dental Hospital of Manchester, Higher Cambridge Street, Manchester M15 6FH
*Correspondence to : Stephen Davies, 73 Buxton Rd, High Lane, Stockport SK6 8DR
email: stephen.j.davies@man.ac.uk

Many of the factors governing the developing occlusion have already been covered in the section on orthodontics, but there are specific instances in which the dentist in general practice will be faced with decisions which could have an influence on the occlusion of child patients. This section aims to present these situations and give guidelines, which will help the reader make the most appropriate treatment decision for their individual patients.

PROBLEMS AND CHOICES:

Premature loss of a tooth in the primary dentition:

If a primary tooth is lost prematurely, then consideration of an extra (balancing) extraction will be necessary.[1,2] This will be with a view to preventing a shift of the midline or resultant disruption of the developing occlusion.

- If a *primary incisor* tooth is lost as a result of caries or trauma this does not usually have an effect on the developing occlusion. Space closure is not going to occur as primary incisor teeth usually become spaced prior to exfoliation.
- If a *primary canine* tooth needs to be extracted, then the contralateral primary canine should also be extracted, in many cases, to prevent an untoward midline shift. Only if the anterior dentition is spaced should unilateral loss be accepted.
- If a single *primary molar* tooth is unsavable and the other teeth have a good prognosis there is no need to extract other molar teeth.

If primary first and/or primary second molars *in three quadrants* have to be extracted

then the equivilant molar in the fourth quadrant should be extracted in order to keep the development and drift symmetrical in each quadrant.

The 'submerging E'

The sight of a primary second molar that appears to be 'submerging' below the level of the occlusal plane of the adjacent teeth is not uncommon. Submergence is an inaccurate term as it is the adjacent teeth which are erupting normally, whilst the *ankylosed* primary molar is remaining static (Fig. 1).

The significance of the 'submerging E' lies not just with the loss of occlusal contact with the opposing teeth, but also the loss of contact, interdentally, with the adjacent teeth, especially distally with the first permanent molar.[3] Figure 2 shows that the first permanent molar has tilted mesially, because of the loss of an effective stabilising contact with the second primary molar.

The issues, therefore, are:
Is there an effective contact with the opposing

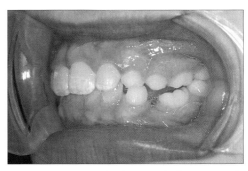

Fig. I **A case where the degree of submergence is minor; there is no tilting of the first permanent molar. This requires no treatment because the primary tooth is usually eventually shed, as long as the permanent sucessor is present**

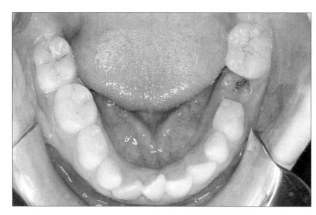

Fig. 2 The submergence of the primary molar is more severe than that in Figure 1. As a consequence the primary second molar has lost contact against the adjacent first permanent molar, which has tilted mesially

teeth and has the first permanent molar started to tilt mesially?

If the 'submerging primary tooth is disrupting the occlusion and there is a permanent successor then the ankylosed primary molar must be extracted to facilitate the eruption of the permanent tooth. There is an argument that this tooth should be extracted even if there is no permanent successor, because the 'submerged E' is not adding to the occlusion and the tilting of the first permanent molar is still an unwanted side effect.

'Firm upper C'

The permanent canine is an essential tooth to consider in the developing occlusion. In an 'ideal' adult occlusion this tooth provides the anterior guidance during an excursive movement of the mandible.

At 9.5 years of age an assessment must be made for the position of the permanent canines.

This is initially done by palpating for the buccal canine bulge.[4] When canines are not palpable the assessment must now include radiographs, for example parallax periapical views. If the canines are veering off from the normal path of eruption the primary canines should be extracted in order to encourage their permanent successors to erupt in the correct position. The eruption of the permanent canines should be reassessed radiographically after 6 months. If their position is not improving referral to a specialist orthodontist is advised.

At ages 9.5 to 10.5 continuing assessment must be made for the canine position. If one primary canine is mobile but the other is firm and the permanent canine is palpable under the mucosa the firm primary canine should be extracted to allow eruption of the successor.

At ages 10.5 onwards if a primary canine is still firm and the permanent canine is **not** palpable under the mucosa the appropriate treatment will depend upon the position of the unerupted canine. Specialist orthodontic opin-

ion should be sought so that an early decision can be taken as to whether:

- To encourage eruption of the permanent successor
- To leave the permanent canine unerupted
- To arrange surgical removal of the unerupted permanent canine

These are treatments that will, almost certainly, require specialist opinion and action; the important element is *timing* and it is only the patient's regular dentist who can ensure a timely referral is made by meticulous monitoring.

Premature loss of a first permanent molar

The literature is replete with data on how to, whether to, or whether not to restore carious first permanent molars, and the debate is still active. The authors consider that a clinician should think carefully before filling and especially before refilling a first permanent molar tooth in a child who is *less than 10 years of age*.[5]

'Restoration at all costs' may not always be the best option. Early extraction of first permanent molars with a poor long-term prognosis may be the best treatment option and must be considered at the outset. The essential question that general dental practitioners need to ask themselves at this time is whether the patient may require orthodontic treatment or will the affected tooth need a crown in the future? If either is likely, then consideration should be given to extraction of the decayed/hypoplastic tooth and also the other first permanent molars. With the welcome arrival of a more restorative treatment expectation in the minds of both the profession and general public, there is a real danger that some dentists may be tempted into restoring severely carious or hypoplastic first permanent molars in their young patients without considering how these teeth fit into the long-term treatment plan. Patients will almost certainly wish to avoid extraction, and whilst supporting this as a general principle, it may fall to the dentist to explain sensitively that this is an instance when extraction is preferable. To compound the problem, if there is a strong indication that if one or two first permanent molars need to be extracted, then extraction of the others must also be considered.

It is our aim to give some guidelines to the treatment planning of these cases. As always the treatment planning starts with an examination.

Examination procedures
Radiographic examination
- Extent of caries
  - Danger of pulpal involvement
  - Sign of caries on smooth surfaces
  - Likelihood of refilling or crown

- Presence of all other unerupted permanent teeth , especially second premolars
- Development of the second permanent molars.

    If an assessment reveals that spontaneous space closure is desirable, timing of extractions is crucial. When the bifurcation of the second molars is visible (just formed) on radiographs and the upper lateral incisor teeth have erupted, this is the best time to extract the first molars to ensure maximum spontaneous alignment. This is because if this stage of development has been reached the lower second molars will move bodily mesially during eruption rather than tilt mesially, which is what happens if extraction are left until later.[6]
- Hypoplasia of unerupted premolar teeth
    If the premolar teeth are of poor quality and there is potential crowding then the balance swings towards conservation of the first permanent molars. The decision on which teeth to extract is delayed until the premolars can be assessed upon their eruption.
- Crowding in the premolar region
    If the first molars are so carious or hypoplastic as to warrant extraction, then often the second primary molars may well have previously been extracted. This may have allowed the first molars to have drifted mesially resulting in a lack of space for the unerupted second premolar. In this situation, extraction of the permanent first molars is certainly indicated as it removes a tooth with a poor prognosis and also relieves premolar crowding (Fig. 3).

Factors influencing decision to extract
- Number of other carious teeth
- Extent of caries (extract if there is pulpal involvement)
- Oral heath status
- Motivation towards dental health
- Presence of malocclusion
- Motivation towards orthodontic treatment

'Restoration at all costs' may not always be the best option

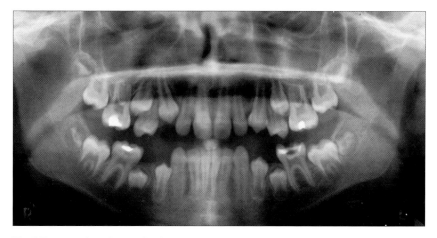

Fig. 3 Panoramic radiograph: the lower first permanent molars are carious and there is premolar crowding

Fig. 4a–c Extraction of first permanent molars. After carrying out the examination, the difficult decision of whether to advise extraction of one or more of the first permanent molars must be taken. The flowcharts in Figures 4 a, b, and c are offered as guidelines, when considering extraction of first permanent molars in patients in the age range of 8 to 10 years.

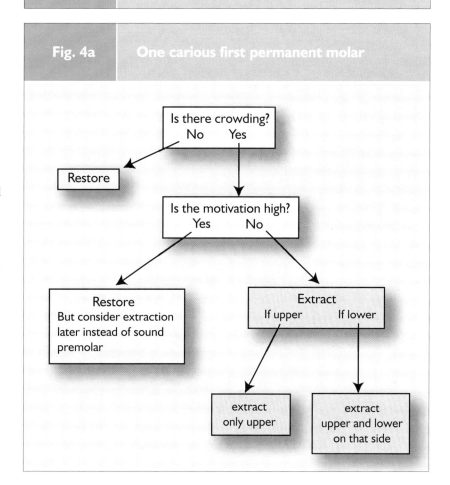

Fig. 4a   One carious first permanent molar

A clinical guide to occlusion

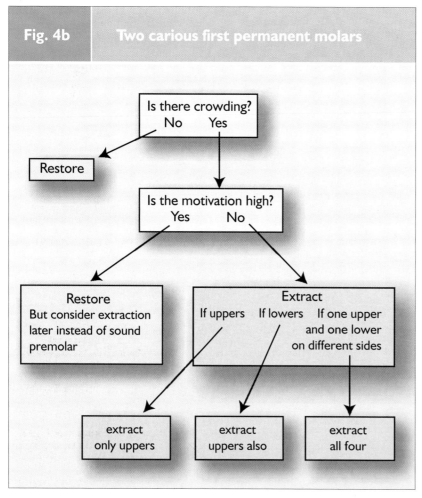

Fig. 4b — Two carious first permanent molars

Is there crowding?
No   Yes

Restore

Is the motivation high?
Yes   No

Restore
But consider extraction
later instead of sound
premolar

Extract
If uppers   If lowers   If one upper
and one lower
on different sides

extract
only uppers

extract
uppers also

extract
all four

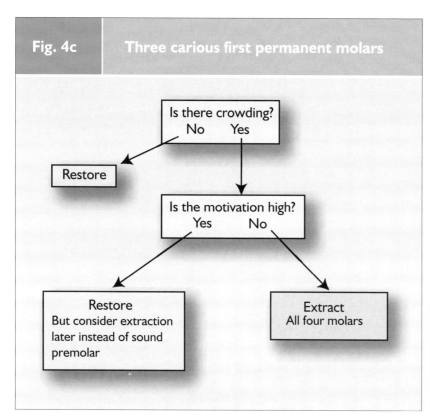

Fig. 4c — Three carious first permanent molars

Is there crowding?
No   Yes

Restore

Is the motivation high?
Yes   No

Restore
But consider extraction
later instead of sound
premolar

Extract
All four molars

Trauma in the permanent dentition

The general dental practitioner frequently encounters a patient presenting with a fractured or avulsed upper incisor tooth. The management of the clinical condition of the fractured, or avulsed, tooth is the subject of many publications and the practical and definitive treatment plan can be sought elsewhere. What we aim to address in this section is the *effect of the treatment plan upon the occlusion.*

Avulsed tooth
• If the avulsed upper tooth is successfully replanted
   There is likely to be no lasting effect upon the developing occlusion, except that effects of the orthodontic treatment on this tooth are likely to be unpredictable, in respect of root resorption.
• If the avulsed upper incisor tooth is not replanted
   A space maintainer should be fitted. The design of this is important from an occlusal point of view. A simple tissue borne spoon denture is not sufficient, because if the prosthetic tooth fractures off from this type of denture then immediately the teeth on either side will start to drift into the space. A more desirable approach is to fit what is in effect an orthodontic appliance with a tooth attached. This design should include clasps on the posterior teeth and stops on

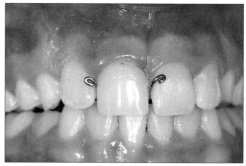

Fig. 5 Anterior view of space maintainer showing mesial and distal stops

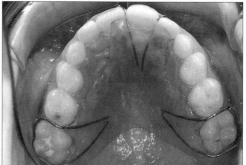

Fig. 6 Mirror view of space maintainer

the teeth either side of the gap, at the level of the gingival papillae. If the tooth fractures off this appliance, then the stops will maintain the space until the appliance can be repaired (Fig. 5, 6).

Fracture of permanent upper incisor
- The most common fracture involves the mesial or distal aspects of the crown. These teeth can be relatively easily and quickly restored by acid etch composite tips so preserving the contact point with the adjacent tooth. The restoration of the contact with the adjacent tooth is very important. In the case illustrated (Fig. 7 a,b) the failure to do so has resulted not only in a mesial and labial tilting of the unrestored tooth, but also in a loss of palatal width. As a consequence of this inaction the restoration of this young patient's dentition represents a major orthodontic and restorative challenge.
- Fortunately a horizontal fracture of the crown of a tooth is less common. It is important that the crown of a tooth so fractured is restored to its original size and shape to prevent occlusal problems developing. The results of this type of injury to the tooth remaining unrestored are over-eruption of the opposing tooth, and less obviously the damaged tooth may tilt buccally because there is reduced lip control.

Missing permanent teeth
In the case of the congenital absence of permanent teeth, the general practitioner's responsibility is early detection. The responsibility, now, for treatment planning lies with the paediatric dentist and specialist orthodontist because with timely referral many of the potential problems of hypodontia can be avoided.

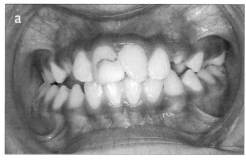

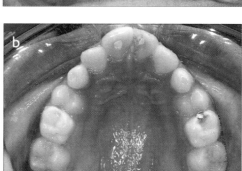

Fig. 7a Despite the poor aesthetics and marginal adaptation, the fracture of UR1 (11) has been restored. The lack of restoration of UL1 (21) has allowed mesial and labial tilting

Fig. 7b The tilting of UL1 (21) has resulted in narrowing of the space for the crown of the tooth

1 Andlaw R J, Rock W P. *A manual of paediatric dentistry.* 4th edn. Edinburgh: Churchill Livingstone, 1996.
2 Ball I A. Balancing the extraction of primary teeth: a review. *Int J Paed Dent* 1993; 4: 176-185.
3 Shaw W C. *Orthodontic and occlusal management.* Oxford: Wright, 1993.
4 British Orthodontic Society. *Young practitioners guide to orthodontics.* British Orthodontic Society, 1998.
5 Blinkhorn A S, Mackie I C. *Treatment planning for paedodontic patients.* London: Quintessence, 1992
6 Mackie I C, Blinkhorn A S, Davies P J H. The extraction of permanent first molars during the mixed dentition period — a guide to treatment planning. *J Paed Dent* 1989; 5: 85-92.

Guidelines of good occlusal practice

1. The examination of the patient involves the teeth, periodontal tissues and articulatory system.
2. There is no such thing as an intrinsically bad occlusal contact, only an intolerable number of times to parafunction on it.
3. The patient's occlusion should be recorded, before any treatment is started.
4. Compare the patient's occlusion against the benchmark of ideal occlusion.
5. A simple, two dimensional means of recording the patient's occlusion before, during and after treatment is an aid to good occlusal practice.
6. The conformative approach is the safest way of ensuring that the occlusion of a restoration does not have potentially harmful consequences.
7. Ensuring that the occlusion conforms (to the patient's pre-treatment state) is a product of examination, design, execution and checking (EDEC)
8. The 'reorganised approach' involves firstly the establishment of a 'more ideal' occlusion in the patient's pretreatment teeth or provisional restorations; and then adhering to that design using the techniques of the 'conformative approach'
9. An 'ideal occlusion' in removable prosthodontics is one which reduced de-stabilising forces
10. The occlusal objective of orthodontic treatment is not clear, but a large discrepancy between centric occlusion and centric relation should not be an outcome of treatment
11. An 'orthodontic' examination of the occlusion should include: the dynamic occlusion; and the jaw relationship in which the patient has centric occlusion
12. The occlusion of periodontally compromised teeth should be designed to reduce the forces to be within the adaptive capabilities of the damaged periodontia
13. **Good occlusal practice in children is determined by the needs of the developing occlusion, consequentially 'restoration at all costs' may not be the best policy.**

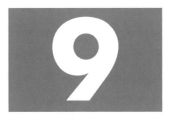

9

Management of tooth surface loss

S. J. Davies,[1] R. J. M. Gray,[2] and A. J. E. Qualtrough,[3]

This chapter is devoted to tooth surface loss *not* caused by caries or trauma. The management of this form of generalised tooth surface loss is included in this series because knowledge of occlusion is needed for both the diagnosis and, when indicated, treatment. There are, however, many other factors involved in the management of generalised tooth surface loss other than those associated with 'occlusion'. These will also be discussed.

The aim of this section is to aid the reader to:
- **Recognise when tooth surface loss is pathological**
- **Determine the aetiology of tooth surface loss**
- **Help the patient to decide whether treatment is indicated**
- **Devise an orderly framework for the design of treatment plans**
- **Provide a rationale for treatment of difficult cases.**

Tooth Surface Loss

**physiological?
pathological?**

[1]*GDP, 73 Buxton Rd, High Lane, Stockport SK6 8DR; P/T Lecturer in Dental Practice, University Dental Hospital of Manchester, Higher Cambridge St., Manchester M15 6FH; [2]Honorary Fellow, University Dental Hospital of Manchester, Higher Cambridge St., Manchester M15 6FH [3]Senior Lecturer and Honorary Consultant in Restorative Dentistry, University Dental Hospital of Manchester, Higher Cambridge St., Manchester M15 6FH
*Correspondence to : Stephen Davies, 73 Buxton Rd, High Lane, Stockport SK6 8DR
email: stephen.j.davies@man.ac.uk

Is the tooth surface loss physiological or pathological?

Tooth surface loss (TSL) may be purely *physiological* (Fig. 1) and occurs as a natural consequence of ageing.[1] Several factors, however, including erosion, abrasion and attrition can render tooth surface loss *pathological* (Fig. 2). As a result of this, symptoms *may* develop and treatment *may* be indicated. Although this chapter will deal with only pathological tooth surface loss, it is important to be able to recognise when tooth surface loss is purely physiological; it cannot be assumed that all tooth surface loss is pathological.

Criteria of physiological tooth surface loss

There appears to be no consensus as to what constitutes physiological tooth surface loss. It would be of assistance to practising dentists if such criteria could be established. In the absence of accepted criteria of physiological tooth surface loss, those of pathological tooth surface loss are presented in Figure 2.

Classification of tooth surface loss

There are usually considered to be three reasons for non carious tooth surface loss. Abfractions should also be considered to be a cause of non-carious TSL.

1. Erosion

Erosion is a chemical process in which the tooth surface is removed in the absence of plaque.[2] Erosive factors may be either intrinsic or extrinsic. Extrinsic sources include drinks such as fresh fruit juices, carbonated drinks, cordials and alcoholic beverages; and some foods and industrial processes. Intrinsic sources include gastro-oesophageal reflux and eating disorders, amongst others.

2. Abrasion

External agents which have an abrasive effect on the teeth include toothbrush bristles and dietary factors.

3. Attrition

Attrition is a process in which tooth tissue is removed as a result of opposing tooth surfaces contacting during function or parafunction. Such direct contact occurs at proximal areas, on supporting cusps and on guiding surfaces during empty grinding movements.

4. Abfractions (stress lesions)

It has been suggested that the stress lesion or abfraction is a consequence of eccentric forces on the natural dentition.[3,4] The theory pro-

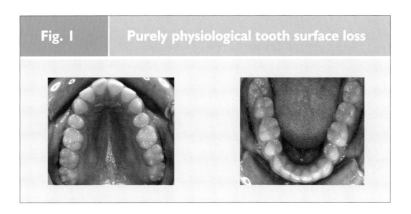

Fig. I   **Purely physiological tooth surface loss**

A clinical guide to occlusion

Fig. 2	Pathological tooth surface loss may result in one or more of the following

- Change in appearance of teeth
- Pain and/or sensitivity
- Loss in occlusal vertical dimension
- Loss in posterior occlusal stability resulting in
  - ◆ Increased tooth wear
  - ◆ Mechanical failure of teeth or restorations
  - ◆ Hypermobility and drifting

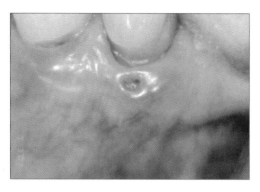

Fig. 3 Abfraction

Terminology:

Function
a normal movement

Parafunction
a normal movement at an abnormal frequency

Dysfunction
an abnormal movement

pounds tooth fatigue, flexure and deformation via biomechanical loading of the tooth structure, primarily at the cervical regions. Cusp flexure causes stress at the cervical fulcrum and results in loss of the overlying tooth structure. The lesion is typically wedge-shaped with sharp line angles, but occlusal abfractions may present as circular invaginations. The magnitude of tooth tissue loss depends on the size, duration, direction, frequency and location of the forces. It should be remembered that abfractive lesions are caused by flexure and fatigue of susceptible teeth at sites that are usually distant from the point of loading. Other factors, such as erosion and abrasion may play a significant role in tooth tissue loss, but the initial force is the biomechanical loading.

Figure 3 shows a cervical cavity which is significantly subgingival and interestingly has caused a fenestration of the overlying attached gingiva. It is highly likely, because of the protection of the overlying soft tissue, that this lesion is an abfraction without any abrasive or erosive component.

Bruxism

What is 'Bruxism'?
Bruxism is an important factor related to tooth surface loss. It is defined as the grinding of teeth during non functional movements of the masticatory system: it is a mandibular parafunction. The wear is usually uniform when opposing teeth are affected. If bruxism is severe, either marked wear of occlusal surfaces will occur or, in cases of compromised periodontal

support, tooth mobility may result. Bruxism can also be associated with muscle spasm, fractured teeth and restorations.[5]

What are the signs of *active* bruxism?
Tooth surface loss or tooth wear cannot be taken as a sign that the patient is an active bruxist. Even if the cause of the TSL was bruxism the patient may no longer be bruxing. The signs of *active* bruxism are tongue scalloping and cheek ridging.[6]

What causes bruxism?
Two aetiological models have been proposed:

(i) *The structural model,* which is based upon the role played by malocclusion or by an alteration in maxillo-mandibular relationship.

(ii) *The functional model,* which highlights the effects of physiological stress as a predominant cause.

There are, however, no reliable predictive indicators to suggest a simple relationship between the causes and effects of bruxism. It was once thought that 'Type A personalities' were more susceptible to stress related bruxism, but current teaching discounts this classification as a gross oversimplification and it is no longer generally used.

Physiological tooth wear
As proximal contacts wear in a normal dentition, there is a compensatory occlusal adjustment. This may happen naturally if the diet is abrasive ie this is as a result of function, not parafunction, and so should not be considered pathological tooth surface loss caused by bruxism.

How can bruxism be treated?
It has been found that the signs and symptoms of bruxism often disappear when occlusal therapy is aimed at the provision of an ideal occlusion: that is the careful elimination of interferences in the static and dynamic occlusion and the maximal distribution of occlusal load. *Occlusal therapy should only be carried out after successful stabilisation splint usage,* and careful 'mock' equilibration on accurately mounted study models. The need for a period of splint therapy is reinforced by the fact that strong clenching has the effect of compressing the periodontal ligament and rebound may take more than half an hour. This is of particular significance when the occlusion is either being assessed or equilibrated.

Furthermore, if the aim is to discourage a bruxist habit, this may be achieved by the patient's intermittent use of an occlusal splint; a stabilisation splint or a localised occlusal interference splint, or in some cases[5] a soft bite guard.

Fig. 4	Initial examination for a patient with tooth surface loss

Patient _____ Date _____ Age _____

1 Is tooth surface loss

Normal ☐
Excessive ☐
Extreme ☐
for a patient of this age?

Is there any evidence that it is progressive?

None ☐
Weak ☐
Strong ☐

2 The following features suggest an aetiology of

EROSION ☐

ABRASION ☐

ATTRITION ☐

_____
_____
_____
_____

3 Known dietary habit? ☐ _____

Known gastric reflux? ☐ _____

Known parafunction? ☐ _____

Other [specify]? ☐ _____

4 Has dento-alveolar compensation taken place? ☐

5 QUALTY OF LIFE ISSUES

Patient is worried about: Appearance ☐

Tooth sensitivity ☐   Tooth or restoration fracture ☐

Soft tissue comfort ☐   Loosening teeth ☐

6 RECORDS taken and TESTS made

Centric Relation jaw registration ☐   Models ☐

Photographs ☐   Tooth measurements taken ☐

Ethyl chloride ☐

Technique

Examination

The patient for whom a diagnosis of pathological tooth surface loss is suspected, should be given a particular examination (Fig. 4).This is in addition to the normal examination of the articulatory system.

This examination is designed to:

- Aid in distinguishing between physiological and pathological T.S.L.
- Reveal any features which may indicate the aetiology
- Indicate whether or not treatment should be carried out
- Highlight any potential difficulties anticipated in treatment.

Is the tooth surface loss pathological?

This question gives rise to Box 1 of the examination sheet (Fig. 4)

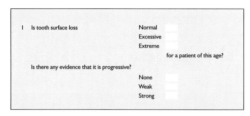

The features of pathological tooth surface loss:
Pathological tooth surface loss may result in a change in the appearance of teeth, considered to be excessive with respect to the age of the patient (Fig. 5).[7]

There may be:

- Sensitivity to thermal stimuli
- A loss in vertical height
- A history of frequent fracture of teeth or restorations
- Hypermobility and drifting.

Are there any features of tooth surface loss which suggest a particular aetiology?

This question gives rise to Boxes 2 and 3 of the examination sheet (Fig. 4)

The features of different types of tooth surface loss

Despite the multi-factorial aetiology of tooth surface loss, certain clinical features may suggest a major contributory factor. Flattening of cusps or incisal edges and localised facets on occlusal or palatal surfaces would indicate a primarily attritional aetiology. Traditionally, cervical lesions caused purely by abrasion have sharply defined margins and a smooth, hard surface. The lesion may become more rounded and shallow if there is an element of erosion present. Once dentine is exposed, the clinical appearance is determined by the relative contribution of the aetiological factors. If wear is primarily attritional, then dentine tends to wear at the same rate as the surrounding enamel. Erosive lesions cause 'cupping' to form in the dentine. When erosion affects the palatal surfaces of upper maxillary teeth, there is often a central area of exposed dentine surrounded by a border

---

Fig. 5

Fig. 5a shows a young patient (18 years), who needs treatment, whereas in Fig. 5b a similar amount of TSL in an older (75years) patient does not necessarily warrant intervention. The patient in Fig. 5c is 45 years old and his request for treatment is justified

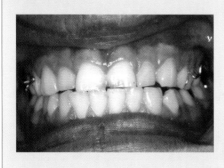
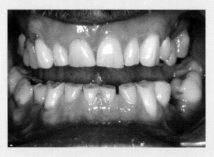
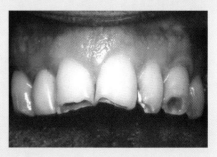

of unaffected enamel.[8]

What are the effects of tooth surface loss?

> 4 Has dento-alveolar compensation taken place?

This question gives rise to Box 4 of the examination sheet (Fig. 4).

The effects of tooth surface loss: Physiological tooth surface loss is normal and results in a reduction in both vertical tooth height and horizontal tooth width.

In physiological tooth surface loss, vertical dimension is maintained by alveolar bone remodelling resulting in an elongation of the (dento-)alveolar process, similarly proximal wear is compensated by a constant forward pressure maintaining tooth to tooth contact.

If pathological vertical tooth surface loss has occurred then there is the possibility that a compensatory growth ('dento-alveolar compensation') may have occurred to some degree. This is an important consideration.

Dento-alveolar compensation

If tooth surface loss affecting the occlusal surfaces of the teeth has occurred, then one might expect to see a reduction in occlusal face height (vertical dimension of occlusion or VDO); or, expressed in a different way, an increase in the freeway space (FWS) could be anticipated. This may be further complicated by forward posturing of the mandible. It is often observed, however, that despite overall tooth surface loss, the freeway space and the resting facial height appear to remain unaltered primarily because of dento-alveolar compensation.

This is important with respect to patient assessment. If restoration of worn teeth is being planned then the *extent of dento-alveolar compensation* would appear to determine the dentist's strategy; defining the need to carry out measures such as crown lengthening, to ensure the same VDO and FWS .

Nevertheless, the fundamental question is:

'Does it matter if the patient's VDO is increased during the restoration of the tooth surface loss (ie the FWS is reduced)?'

The answer is different for each patient. No occlusion can be said to be 'wrong' rather it is the case that in certain patients, at particular times in their lives, some occlusal patterns will not be tolerated. An occlusion can only be judged by the reaction of the tissues surrounding it, so it is with the issue of an increase in VDO.

In the case of a patient presenting with some dento-alveolar compensation, the clinician should assess whether or not that patient can tolerate an increased VDO (reduced FWS) by the construction of a stabilisation splint and/or provisional restorations.

The incidence of dento-alveolar compensation

It has been observed that in the normal adult dentition, the FWS remains constant and even in those patients who exhibit significant tooth surface loss the VDO is unaffected in 80% and a normal FWS of 3 mm is exhibited. If treatment of a patient within this group is necessary then crown lengthening procedures may be indicated. This will enable adequate reduction of the teeth at crown preparation so allowing the same VDO to be maintained. Alternatively restoration of the patient's dentition may be provided at an increased VDO (reduced FWS). Some may argue that any increase in FWS should be proportionate to the degree of attrition.

Does the patient want/need treatment ?

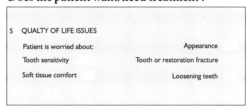

This question gives rise to Box 5 of the examination sheet (Fig. 4)

Patient's wants and needs

It is essential as in all areas of clinical practice to carefully consider the patient's anxieties and desires in addition to the clinical features before advice is given.

Monitoring

Monitoring involves taking a series of repeated examinations and certain measurements over a period of time in order to assess whether a condition is progressive. Monitoring is essential in the management of tooth surface loss.

In the literature several methods of assessing tooth wear have been described including:

- General assessment of extracted teeth,
- Chemical analysis
- Physical methods (polarised light/indentation techniques/profilometry) scanning electron microscopic analysis
- Digital image analysis.

These are research tools and are not applicable to clinical practice. Therefore, a monitoring protocol to assess tooth surface loss is presented (Fig. 6a,b). It is easy to use and by this method it is easy to record the progression of tooth surface loss.

Monitoring is, of course, only an option when baseline measurements have been taken. This emphasises the need for the dentist to examine and record tooth surface loss. To facilitate this a protocol for the *initial*

Fig. 6a	Tooth surface loss monitoring

Patient

Date

Age

Primary aetiology

EROSION

ABRASION

ATTRITION

RV no: DATE OF LAST RV INTERVAL

AFFECTED TEETH

Tooth surface loss

Dentine exposed
1 Mild, 2 Moderate
3 Severe

Sensitivity
(pt's c/o)

Tooth mobility
Cl I, II, Cl III

Fractured/Failed
restorations

Hairline fracture
lines

OTHER NOTES

Page 1 of 2

Fig. 6b	Tooth surface loss monitoring

Patient   Date

OTHER SIGNS

Active bruxism?   Tongue scalloping

                       Cheek ridging

T.M.J. exam   Noise

                       Range of motion

        Tenderness to palpitation

Muscle tenderness

RECORDS TAKEN

Photographs   Impressions

Measurements from A.D.J.

ASSESSMENT at this time

Non-progressive

Maybe progressive [not marked and no symptoms]

Progressive [obvious]

Progressive [obvious and symptomatic]

TREATMENT at this time

Page 2 of 2

examination of a patient with TSL has been presented (Fig. 4).

Treatment

The key question to be answered is:

> '*Does this patient need treatment?*'

There are no hard and fast rules and the need for treatment should be established after considering:

- The degree of wear relative to the age of the patient
- The aetiology
- The symptoms
- The patient's wishes.

Treatment may be either passive or active

Passive treatment

Monitoring (Figs 6a and 6b)

This has already been discussed under the 'Examination section' and it represents a review process. Monitoring is the only way in which TSL can be assessed as being active or static. It is, therefore, the case that in most situations a period of monitoring should be carried out prior to considering active treatment.

Prevention

This is 'treatment' of *future* tooth surface loss. If the extent of existing tooth surface loss is considered to be acceptable, the appropriate treatment is clearly to try to prevent further TSL, which could render the patient needing restorative treatment. The form of the preventive treatment will be dependent on the aetiology of the TSL, so determining the cause is essential.

For a patient whose tooth surface loss is essentially caused by *erosive fluids,* advice regarding diet, the use of sugar free chewing gum, and the prescription of a fluoride mouthwash will almost certainly be indicated. It may be also necessary to liaise with the doctor if you suspect the patient suffers from a depressive illness.

If the wear is primarily caused by *abrasion* then examination and modification of the tooth cleaning habits will be indicated.

If the wear is caused by *attrition,* then the patient should be advised of any possible bruxist habits. The provision of one of three different sorts of splints could be considered. A soft bite guard can help in breaking a bruxist habit or simply will protect the teeth during the bruxist habit. A localised occlusal interference splint is designed to break the bruxist habit, and can be worn easily during the day. A stabilisation splint reduces bruxism by providing an ideal occlusion: it also enables the clinician to locate and record centric relation.[9]

Active treatment

Non-carious loss of tooth tissue may require treatment for one or more of the following reasons:

- Sensitivity
- Aesthetics
- Function
- Space loss in the vertical dimension.

The latter may present a critical problem and both the need for restorative treatment and the complexity of that restorative treatment may depend upon whether or not dento-alveolar compensation has occurred, as previously discussed.

Where do we start?

Careful planning regarding the reconstruction of a worn dentition is essential and, as in any other restorative treatment plan, the first decision to be made is whether or not the restorations will be designed to:

- Harmonise with the existing occlusion ie the *conformative approach,* or
- Make a change towards an ideal occlusion ie the *reorganised approach.*

The conformative approach

The following criteria should be met if the conformative approach is to be considered:

1 The patient has an ideal occlusion, with centric occlusion occurring in centric relation, and the anterior guidance is at the front of the mouth. (This is not a common finding)
2 The patient does not have an ideal occlusion. However, the teeth to be restored are not deflecting contacts (those contacts which guide the mandible into their centric occlusion).
3 It is not predicted that any other teeth in the mouth will need to be restored because of further tooth surface loss.
4 There is no temporomandibular disorder.

The reorganised approach

If these criteria do not pertain, then a re-organised approach will need to be considered.

Management of a patient with pathological tooth surface loss

Treat or monitor?

Whether or not a particular patient exhibiting TSL needs treatment or monitoring can only be determined by a complex series of decisions. An attempt to illustrate this process, relatively simply, is presented as Fig. 7.

Options for patient needing treatment

The alternatives are equally complex for treatment if the decision has been taken that a patient needs treatment.

The process starts with an examination of the jaw relationship in which the patient is presently occluding (does CO occur in CR?).

From that decision it is possible to provide some structure to the treatment planning

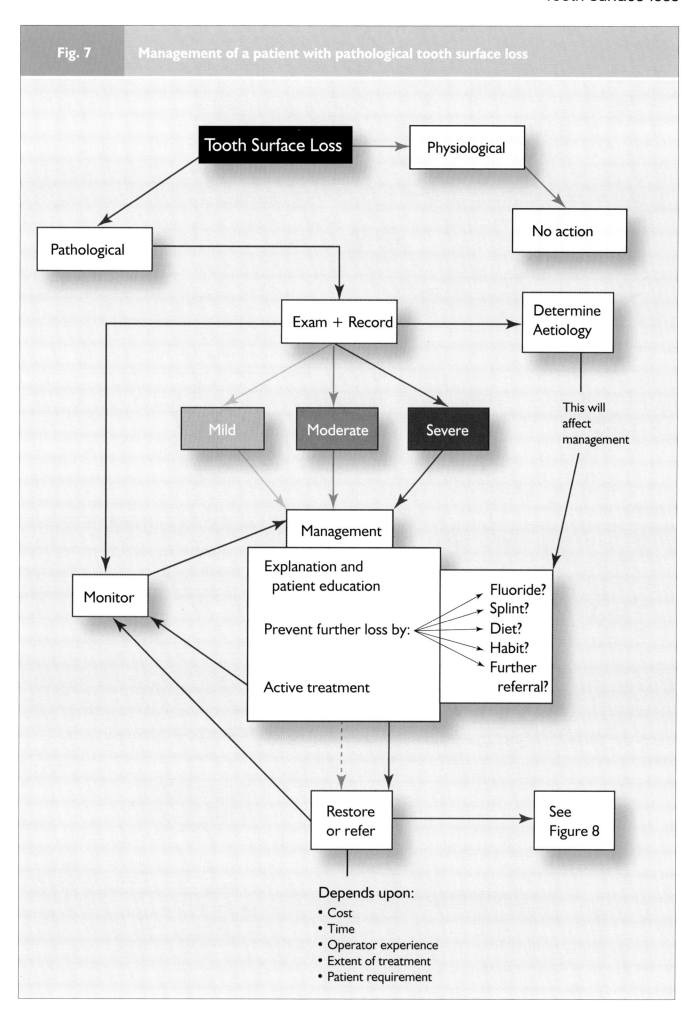

Fig. 7   Management of a patient with pathological tooth surface loss

A clinical guide to occlusion

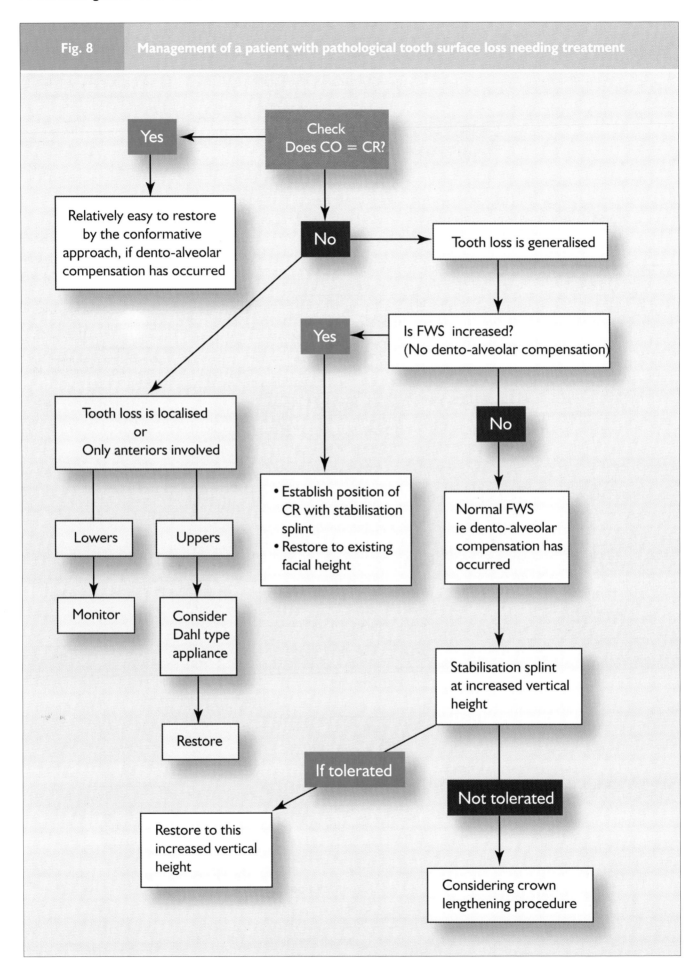

Fig. 8   Management of a patient with pathological tooth surface loss needing treatment

Check
Does CO = CR?

Yes

Relatively easy to restore by the conformative approach, if dento-alveolar compensation has occurred

No

Tooth loss is generalised

Is FWS increased?
(No dento-alveolar compensation)

Yes

Tooth loss is localised
or
Only anteriors involved

No

- Establish position of CR with stabilisation splint
- Restore to existing facial height

Normal FWS
ie dento-alveolar compensation has occurred

Lowers

Uppers

Monitor

Consider Dahl type appliance

Restore

Stabilisation splint at increased vertical height

If tolerated

Not tolerated

Restore to this increased vertical height

Considering crown lengthening procedure

	Guidelines of good occlusal practice

1   The examination of the patient involves the teeth, periodontal tissues and articulatory system.

2   There is no such thing as an intrinsically bad occlusal contact, only an intolerable number of times to parafunction on it.

3   The patient's occlusion should be recorded, before any treatment is started.

4   Compare the patient's occlusion against the benchmark of ideal occlusion.

5   A simple, two dimensional means of recording the patient's occlusion before, during and after treatment is an aid to good occlusal practice.

6   The conformative approach is the safest way of ensuring that the occlusion of a restoration does not have potentially harmful consequences.

7   Ensuring that the occlusion conforms (to the patient's pre-treatment state) is a product of examination, design, execution and checking (EDEC)

8   The 'reorganised approach' involves firstly the establishment of a 'more ideal' occlusion in the patient's pretreatment teeth or provisional restorations; and then adhering to that design using the techniques of the 'conformative approach'

9.   An 'ideal occlusion' in removable prosthodontics is one which reduces de-stabilising forces

10. The occlusal objective of orthodontic treatment is not clear, but a large discrepancy between centric occlusion and centric relation should not be an outcome of treatment

11. An 'orthodontic' examination of the occlusion should include: the dynamic occlusion; and the jaw relationship in which the patient has centric occlusion

12. The occlusion of periodontally compromised teeth should be designed to reduce the forces to be within the adaptive capabilities of the damaged periodontia

13. Good occlusal practice in children is determined by the needs of the developing occlusion, consequentially 'restoration at all costs' may not be the best policy.

14. **Not all tooth surface loss needs treatment, but effective monitoring is essential**

15. **Dento-alveolar compensation has often occured in patients exibiting marked tooth surface loss.**

1   Flint S, Scully C. Orofacial changes and related disease. *Dent Update* 1988; **15**: 337-342.
2   Milosevic A. Eating disorders and the dentist. *Br Dent J* 1999; **186**: 109-113.
3   Braem M, Lambrechts P, Vanherle G. Stress-induced lesions. *J Prosthet Dent* 1992; **67**: 718-722.
4   Grippo J A. A new classification of hard tissue lesions. *J Aesthetic Dent* 1988; **3**: 14-19.
5   Dawson P E. *Evaluation, diagnosis and treatment of occlusal problems.* St Louis: C V Mosby Co. 2nd ed. 1989, p457.
6   Franks A S T. Masticatory muscle hypertonicity and temporomandibular joint dysfunction. *J Prosthet Dent* 1965; **6**: 1122-1131.
7   Smith B G N, Knight J K. An index for measuring the wear of teeth. *Br Dent J* 1984; **156**: 435-438.
8   Kelleher M, Bishop K. Tooth surface loss: an overview. *Br Dent J* 1999; **186**: 61-66.
9   Gray R M J, Davies S J, Quayle A A. A clinical approach to temporomandibular disorders: Splint therapy. *Br Dent J* 1994; **177**: 135-142.

Good occlusal practice in the provision of implant borne prostheses

S. J. Davies,[1]* R. J. M. Gray,[2] and M. P. J. Young,[3]

The increased use of endosseous dental implants means that many dentists will encounter patients with dental implants in their everyday practice. Dental practitioners might be actively involved in the provision of implant borne prostheses at both the surgical and restorative phases, or only at the restorative stage. This section is written for all dentists and aims to examine the subject of occlusion within implantology. It aims to provide guidelines of good occlusal practice to be used in the design of the prosthesis that is supported or retained by one or more implants.

As implantology is a 'new' discipline of dentistry, there are fewer standard texts and this section, therefore, is much more extensively referenced than the subjects that have been considered to date.

10

In this part, we will discuss:
- **The fundamental principles of implantology**
- **How occlusal factors might influence implant success**
- **General considerations of implant case planning**
- **How to increase the chances of implant success by prescribing an ideal occlusion**

Even those general dental practitioners who are _not_ implant providers are likely in the future to be _responsible for the maintenance_ of implants

---

Implantology is based upon osseointegration

---

[1]*GDP, 73 Buxton Rd, High Lane, Stockport SK6 8DR; P/T Lecturer in Dental Practice, University Dental Hospital of Manchester, Higher Cambridge St., Manchester M15 6FH; [2]Honorary Fellow, University Dental Hospital of Manchester, Higher Cambridge St., Manchester M15 6FH [3]Research Associate, Clinical Academic Group of Oral and Maxillofacial Sciences, University Dental Hospital of Manchester M15 6FH; BUPA Hospital, Whalley Range, Manchester M16 8AJ *Correspondence to : Stephen Davies, 73 Buxton Rd, High Lane, Stockport SK6 8DR email: stephen.j.davies@man.ac.uk

Osseointegration

For osseointegration to occur *predictably* clinical guidelines have been developed to optimise success rates:[1]

- The implant must consist of a suitable biomaterial with appropriate surface properties
- Adequate vital bone must be present to support the implant
- A precise surgical fit must be achieved between the bone and the implant
- The implant must be inserted with a low-trauma technique to avoid overheating of the bone during preparation of the receptor site
- The implant should not be subject to functional loads during a healing period of 3-6 months (This traditional protocol is now being questioned).

Although these guidelines do not mention 'occlusion', once integrated, dental implants must be restored *sympathetically* with due regard to occlusion since unfavourable loading has been cited as a major cause of failure. This chapter will present the factors that influence the occlusal schemes used for prostheses supported or retained by endosseous dental implants. Since relatively few studies have been designed with the sole aim of comparing different occlusal schemes, it is difficult to be certain

what is the best occlusion for a given clinical situation. Current techniques and materials tend to be based on what has evolved over years of clinical practice and laboratory research. They are based on what is believed, rather than what is known, to be good occlusal practice in implantology.

'Osseointegration' is the biological process that results in a close structural relationship between vital bone and a dental implant. Successfully integrated and carefully loaded implants have been shown to be capable of being retained by the host tissues for many years. Osseointegration was first defined as 'the direct structural and functional connection between ordered living bone and the surface of a load carrying implant'.[2] More recently this has been defined as 'a process whereby a clinically asymptomatic rigid fixation of alloplastic materials is achieved and maintained in bone during functional loading'.[3] Obviously, the significant difference between 'osseointegration' and the attachment of teeth to the alveolus is the absence of a periodontal ligament.

Although axons have been identified in peri-implant regions, their functional significance is not clearly understood.[4] At present, the proprioceptive capability of restored implants is usually attributed to bone deformation of the periosteal mechanoreceptors on implant loading.[5] Regardless of the precise mechanism for such proprioception, it has been shown that the threshold of tactile sensitivity is approximately eight times less than that of natural teeth.[6] In addition, the range of 'food-holding' forces for patients with implants is significantly higher than those for patients with natural teeth.[7] When prescribing or modifying occlusal contacts for implant prostheses, it should be borne in mind that the patient's perception of occlusal irregularities and occlusal loads is much reduced and, therefore, should not be solely relied upon.

Current application of oral implants
The current application of implants is much more extensive than when implants were first utilised. In stark contrast to their initial applications [when predominantly only edentulous patients were treated with fixed dentures], implants are now inserted into:

- Partially dentate patients with a healthy or compromised periodontium.
- Posterior regions of the maxilla and mandible
- Sites in which the bone has been augmented.

In addition, many different types of prostheses may now be implant-supported:

- Fixed crowns
- Fixed bridges
- Fixed dentures
- Precision removable dentures
- Removable overdentures (mucosa and implant supported)

Implant success
Criteria for implant success have been outlined some years ago.
There should be an absence of:
- Mobility
- Associated radiolucency
- Pain
- Infection or iatrogenic neuropathies.
- Peri-implant vertical bone loss
  < 1.0 mm in the first year of loading
  < 0.2 mm per annum thereafter.

Implant success vs implant survival
In recent years, 'implant survival' (implant retention at the end-point of the study) appears to be increasingly used when reporting treatment outcomes.[8–17] This term might be mistakenly interpreted as being synonymous with *implant success* as defined above.[18] Criteria for success are not always clearly defined and might be 'system specific'. Since implant survival is a crude measure of implant health, research that uses this term cannot be considered to be as meaningful as

that which defines and measures implant success. Therefore, when evaluating clinical research studies, a critical appraisal must be made.

Despite numerous early studies that reported success rates in excess of 90%, more recently lower success rates have been reported.[19] This might be explained by the use of implants in more demanding circumstances, poor operator technique, or the use of an implant system with an unproven track record. A further factor might be the level of experience of the surgeons that provide implant treatment.[20]

The failing implant
Whilst the efficacy of implants has been amply demonstrated for certain systems, fewer studies are available for any implant system to support their effectiveness in 'real life' studies where, for example, selection criteria might be more relaxed.[21] As for all medical and dental treatments, we can expect the proven effectiveness of implants to be less than their proven efficacy. Against this background, it is important not only to define implant failure, but also to examine how it might be prevented.

A failing implant can be defined as one in which the criteria for success are not met. 'Peri-implant' inflammation (peri-implantitis) presents a similar clinical picture to periodontal inflammation, with bone loss as a key feature. 'Perimucositis', has been reserved for soft tissue infection around an implant, whilst 'perimplantitis' implies accompanying bone loss (classification and review of implant failures).[22–25]

The 'failing' implant often presents as a chronic then terminal condition ultimately leading to implant exfoliation.

The stages of implant failure have been suggested to be (after Newman):[26]

1. Gingival inflammation
2. Gingival hypertrophy
3. Progressive deepening of pockets
4. Progressive attachment loss
5. Progressive bone loss
6. Change in microbial microflora
7. 'Implant deintegration' with mobility and peri-implant radiolucency
8. Implant exfoliation

The suggested aetiological factors for implant failure are:

- Reduced host resistance
- Plaque accumulation
- Occlusal stress
- Systemic factors eg diabetes and smoking

Although a wide range of techniques has been employed to stabilise failing implants, it is recognised that the evidence to support these interventions appears poor at present.[27]

Case responsibility

The determination of case responsibility is an important consideration for two reasons.

Firstly, implants can and do fail and the causes of failure are not completely understood.

Secondly, the provision of an implant borne restoration is often a team effort. If the same clinician carries out both surgical and restorative phases, the responsibility for design and execution of the treatment, together with an appropriate maintenance programme is unequivocal. However, when implant treatment is delivered as a 'team' (at one or more sites) the question of responsibility for implant failure becomes more complex and indeed more contentious. Failure under this regime may result in a debate which does the profession no credit.

When implant therapy is delivered by a 'team', close collaboration between the surgeon, restorative dentist and dental technician is essential. The surgeon must ask for guidance as to the optimal restorative implant location. Equally, the restorative dentist must appreciate the anatomical constraints when giving some guidance on the ideal position with regards to the proposed occlusal platform. The implant technician must have some concept of preferred occlusal schemes if appropriate occlusal contacts are to be incorporated into the implant supported prosthesis. In such situations, it is suggested that the most experienced member of the implant team becomes the 'team-leader', whether they be surgeon or restorative dentist.

The *team leader* must ensure that the joint treatment plan minimises the risk of implant failure. This is particularly important since the current evidence to support the efficacy of implant-rescue techniques is weak. The degree of responsibility will vary according to the experience of the team members, but the principle that a patient's treatment should not suffer through a lack of communication between the clinicians involved is paramount. The 'team leader' is responsible for ensuring that the appropriate communication exists to satisfy the needs of the case.

Occlusal overload as a cause of implant failure

It has been established that trauma from occlusion may be a factor in the aetiology of implant failure.[22–28] It has been suggested that a radiological appearance of "saucerisation or furrowing" is associated with occlusal overload (Fig. 1).[29]

Whereas the natural dentition is capable of physiologically adapting to traumatic occlusions, the absence of a periodontal ligament means that dental implants are more easily overloaded and this can to lead to implant fail-

> **The Surgeon's Tale**
> 'The implants were successfully integrated, but failed because of excess loads'
>
> *or*
>
> **The Restorative Dentist's Tale**
> 'The implants were poorly integrated and so failed under normal masticatory loads'
>
> *either way*
>
> **The Patient's Tale**
> 'My implants have failed !'

ure. Left untreated, an overloaded implant will ultimately exfoliate. Remedial action must be speedily undertaken to redress the unfavourable loading conditions.

The causes of occlusal stress are numerous and include:

- Inadequate number of implants to support the prosthesis fitted
- Heavy occlusal contacts in centric occlusion
- Working-side interferences (as opposed to balanced contacts)
- Non-working side interferences
- Excessive buccal or lingual cantilever (the occlusal table too wide for the implant diameter) (Fig. 5b)

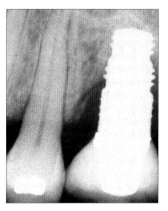

Fig. 1 'Funnelling' or 'Saucerisation': a possible sign of occlusal overload

Technique
Recommendations for occlusal schema for implant supported prostheses

It is the nature of osseointegration that determine the features of an 'ideal' occlusion for an implant supported prosthesis.

The fundamental nature of osseointegration (no periodontal ligament) means that proprioceptive and aptaptive potential is less than with natural teeth:

- The implant is rigidly attached and will move or intrude much less
- Although connection to the central nervous system are believed to exist, it is accepted that proprioception is reduced
- An implant cannot undergo orthodontic movement

An ideal occlusal scheme for fixed implant supported prostheses has been recommended:[30]

- A centric occlusion 'cusp to central fossa' contact which is light
- An ideal anterior guidance: that is canine-guidance or group-function; no posterior interferences
- Axial loading of the implants

Historically, it has been recommended that non-axial loads should be dissipated by the use

> **The absence of a periodontal membrane is believed to be the reason why endosseous implants appear to tolerate non-axial loads poorly**

of inter-implant splinting, by means of bars or fixed-beam structures, and 'double-construction' techniques. However, in recent years this principle has been questioned[31] and multi-implant cases are now being restored as multiple, non-splinted, single teeth implants. This approach, however, is a recent development and the evidence base is correspondingly light. As it is widely acknowledged that the bone of the posterior maxilla is poor in quality, the use of non-splinted, multiple implants restored with fixed prostheses in this region is considered to carry a greater risk of failure. Careful loading in the posterior regions seems especially important to sustain acceptable implant success rates.

To conform or to re-organise?
The decision to provide an occlusion in 'an implant case', either conforming to the pre-existing occlusion or re-organising the occlusion, will be made in exactly the same manner as in any other restoration treatment plan. This decision making process is described earlier.

Two guidelines are paramount:

- If it is possible to follow the conformative approach this is the safest route
- If an occlusion is to be re-organised, establishing and recording Centric Relation is the essential first step.

Classification of osseointegrated prostheses
The key features of an appropriate occlusion will in part depend upon the type of prosthesis. The different types of prostheses will be considered under the following classification:

- Single-tooth implant
- Full-arch, implant supported prosthesis
- Free-standing, fixed-prosthesis Kennedy classes I, II, III, IV
- Implant-retained overdenture
- Implant & tooth-retained, fixed-prosthesis

1. Single tooth replacement by implant retained crown
The single, anterior tooth implant is now an accepted and a highly predictable means of tooth replacement. Until recently, molar tooth replacement by an endosseous dental implant was considered contra-indicated. Prior to the development of 'wide-diameter' implants, molars were restored using two narrow implants. Recent studies indicate that similar success rates can be expected for double or single implant molar replacements.[32–34] A poor occlusal scheme is likely to increase the risk of implant failure in the posterior region, since the chewing forces in this region greatly exceed those in the anterior region, and because bone quality is poorer.

Ideal occlusion for single tooth implant
- Light load (infra-occlusion by 30 μm) under heavy clenching
- Occlusal force directed down the long axis of implant
- Light or no occlusal contact during excentric excursions.

Discussion of requirements of 'ideal' occlusion for single tooth implant (Fig. 2)

1. The occlusion required for the single tooth replacement is similar, but not identical, to the natural dentition. In centric occlusion, the implant supported crown should have a clearance of 30 μm. This clearance is important since the natural teeth can be intruded in their sockets under heavy loads whereas the implant retained prosthesis will not intrude. Any clinician who is used to adjusting their conventional crown and bridgework using shimstock (thickness 8μm) will recognise that 30 μm is a significant clearance. Failure to build in this appropriate occlusal clearance would expose the implant-retained fixed-prosthesis to excessive forces *under heavy loading conditions*. Unfortunately, the patient cannot be relied upon to report that an implant supported crown is 'high' because the absence of a periodontal membrane means that there is limited proprioception in the implant-alveolar bone system.
2. Endosseous implants are best able to withstand forces that are directed down the long axis of the implant, because of the absence of the periodontal ligament sling. This requirement is not purely a consideration in the restorative phase of the treatment, the placing of an implant should wherever possible take account of the eventual occlusal loading.
3. Light excentric contacts are a vital requirement to avoid non-axial loading.

It is possible to 'hide' the implant within the natural occlusion by slight infra-occlusion, so the single tooth implant can easily be protected from mechanical overload. Adjacent natural teeth should be 'recruited' to provide proprioceptive protection from excess loads.

2. Full-arch, implant supported prosthesis
Two occlusal schemes have been described and recommended for the restoration of full-arch implant supported, fixed-prostheses:[35]

1. Mutually protected occlusion (MPO)
2. Lingualized occlusion (LO)

a) Mutually protected occlusion (MPO)
This concept recommends that in centric relation there is only posterior tooth contact. The maxillary palatal cusps and mandibular

buccal cusps should occlude with their opposing occlusal fossae. Thus, anterior teeth positively disclude the posterior teeth in all excentric excursions, protecting the posterior teeth (or implants) from harmful lateral forces. This type of mutually protected occlusion has been reported to be the most efficient in terms of mastication, combined with what is widely regarded to be the optimal aesthetic appearance. This 'gnathological' scheme is believed to closely represent the 'perfect' natural occlusion.

Whereas most of us can describe this type of occlusion, to fabricate, fit and monitor such an occlusion requires considerable laboratory and technical expertise, substantial clinical skills and ample chair-side time. MPO requires that a large number of contacts between the posterior teeth should occur simultaneously. The contacts between the back teeth should be tripodal cusp-to-fossae. Analysing and modifying such complex contacts is generally considered very difficult in full-arch implant supported prostheses. Chairside occlusal equilibriation will almost always be necessary.

Guideline: Avoid non-axial loading whenever possible. Shallow central fossae with tripodal cuspal contacts should be attained. The presence of ridge-lapping should be minimised whenever possible and the distal length of a cantilever has been empirically recommended between 10 and 20 mm. More recently, it has been suggested that the optimal distal cantilever is in the region of just 7 mm. When exceeding this length, clinicians should carefully consider the number, location and precise arrangement supporting implants.[36]

b) Lingualized occlusion (LO)

Since it is acknowledged that MPO is difficult and time-consuming to fabricate, fit and maintain, alternative occlusal schemes have been proposed. Specifically, 'lingualized occlusion' has been recommended for the restoration of full-arch dental implants. The aims are the same but the major benefits of this occlusal scheme are the comparative simplicity with which it can be established and maintained, and its ability to direct masticatory loads axially onto the supporting dental implants.

The key feature is the arrangement of the posterior teeth so that only the *maxillary palatal* cusps (hence: 'lingualized' occlusion; or should it have been called *'palatalised'* occlusion?) occlude with *shallow* mandibular central fossae. There is no contact between the mandibular buccal cusp and palatal maxillary cusps which might result in a inclined (non-axial) contact. Laboratory fabrication time is reduced and this scheme represents a posterior occlusion that can be more readily

Fig. 2	Predictability of success for a single tooth implant

Ideal Case

- Tooth absent UR1
- Aetiology of tooth loss = acute trauma
- Vertical bone loss = nil
- Adequate bone width
- Adequate posterior occlusion
- Absence of prematurities in CR
- Canine-guided disclusion
- Protrusive contact should be evenly distributed on the incisors
- Class I incisor relationship anterior clearance 30 μm in centric occlusion

Predicted Success is Very High
Guideline Conform to existing occlusion which is atraumatic (The Conformative Approach)

Non-Ideal Case

- Tooth absent UR1
- Aetiology of tooth loss: root fracture (previously post-retained crown)
- Vertical bone loss = nil,
- Adequate bone width.
- Severe cuspal attrition of all four canines
- Multiple teeth with mirror-faceting
- Reduced vertical dimension
- Posterior occlusion exhibits very wide based occlusal contacts
- Edge to edge incisor relationship
- Group function exhibited in lateral excursion
- No posterior disclusion in protrusive excursions

Predicted Success is Questionable
Guideline: Existing occlusion is unfavourable and may have contributed to the loss of this tooth, so implant treatment is contra-indicated until the natural occlusion is changed to being a more ideal one (ie the re-organised approach). The alternative is to proceed with implant treatment after making the patient aware that the implant will be placed into a comparatively hostile environment. Certainly if tooth surface loss continues, the implant will become highly susceptible to overload.

observed in both the laboratory and clinical environments thereby enabling any unfavourable occlusal contacts to be identified and corrected more easily.

A very minor disadvantage of lingualized occlusion is the creation, by definition, of a slight buccal space between the buccal cusps of the mandibular teeth and their maxillary counterparts. However, since this spacing occurs in the posterior region of the arches, the aesthetic implications are minimal.

Guideline: Avoid non-axial loading whenever possible. Shallow mandibular central fossae with maxillary palatal cuspal contacts should be attained. The presence of ridge-lapping should be minimised whenever possible and the length of a cantilever should not extend further than 7 mm beyond the most distal implant (See later for an explanation of ridge lapping).

3. Free-standing, fixed-bridges (Kennedy Classes I -IV inclusive)

a) Kennedy Class I
*Guideline: In these **bilateral free end saddle** cases both posterior sections of the arch are restored with osseointegrated bridges. The anterior guidance will be provided by the natural dentition as long as the implant supported bridges are designed to allow adequate posterior disclusion. There is a conflict in the design of these bridges, which is impossible to resolve. On the one hand there is an indication to make the occlusal stops on the **posterior** bridges lighter by about 30 μm than those in the remaining natural teeth. On the other hand, (given that there is general agreement that it is more ideal that the back teeth contact harder than the front teeth) this will not be possible if the posterior occlusion is exclusively provided by the implant supported bridges. It is not unusual for clinicians to have such issues to reconcile. The best treatment outcome is likely to be provided by those clinicians who realise that there is a danger of trauma from occlusion and so will carefully monitor the situation.*

b) Kennedy Class II
Guideline: This clinical situation (unilateral free end saddle) can be regarded as a very favourable application for a fixed prosthesis because the natural teeth will provide the occlusion; whilst the contralateral unilateral free end saddle can be restored with implant supported bridgework that has 30 μm clearance.

c) Kennedy Class III
Guideline: Where there are bounded posterior saddles the use of implants is again ideal because the adjacent natural teeth that bound the edentulous space will allow the construction of the restorations with the 30 μm clearance; and the anterior teeth will provide the ideal anterior guidance.

d) Kennedy Class IV
Guideline: This is an anterior bounded saddle. When there is as a large span (for example UR4 (14) to UL4(24) it is very difficult to restore with a fixed bridge because of the excessive torque that is a result of the cantilever. In contrast, the insertion of four to six anterior implants can easily and predictably treat this situation. The implant-supported Kennedy Class IV bridge must provide an appropriate anterior guidance which achieves posterior disclusion, and a shallow anterior guidance is recommended. In addition, is advisable to prescribe slightly greater freedom in centric occlusion than for natural anterior teeth.

4. Overdentures
Overdentures may be used for both maxillary and mandibular edentulous cases.
Guideline: In the upper arch it is usual to use a minimum of four implants for denture retention and full palatal coverage is employed for additional support and retention. However, in view of the generally softer bone in the maxilla than in the mandible, six implants would be preferable, in order to reduce the functional load on each implant. In the mandible, two implants may be sufficient. The occlusion recommended in either denture is fully balanced lingualized occlusion.

The particular problem of designing an occlusion between a mucosa supported upper complete denture and an implant retained lower complete denture are discussed under 'New combination syndrome' (Section 3C(iii) of the section on Good Occlusal Practice in Removable Prosthodontics)

5. Implant and tooth-retained, fixed-prosthesis
The concept of linking natural teeth to implants to support a fixed bridge has stimulated considerable debate and research. It is widely accepted that this situation is less than ideal since it requires rigid bone-anchored implant(s) to be joined to a relatively mobile natural tooth. The reason why it is extremely difficult to design an ideal occlusion for a fixed bridge that is supported in this way is that the bridge would be a *rigid* link between two totally different attachments to bone. Reaction to occlusal load is dependant upon the form of the attachment to bone. Since the attachments of teeth and implants are so different, *the reaction to occlusal load is bound to differ;* and this can have an adverse effect on the attachments and/or the prosthesis.

The IMZ® (FRIADENT AG, Manheim, Germany) implant system possesses a compressible component that reduces the impact of an occlusal force to the supporting implant.[37] It has been suggested that this 'stress-breaking' feature lends itself to linkage with natural teeth. However, intrusion of the natural supporting tooth has been reported when IMZ implants in combination with natural teeth are used to support fixed bridges.[38] Although this system seems to overcome the inherent problems of linking teeth to implants, it is widely acknowledged that the scientific evidence for this is limited at present. As a consequence, fixed prostheses supported by teeth and implants should be avoided whenever possible.

CONSIDERATIONS OF CASE PLANNING
The relationship between the occlusion and the implant/bone that will support it is extremely important. Restoration by the provision of implant supported prosthesis pre-

Fig. 3

Ridge Lapping

The pattern of bone resorption is not only apical, but also lingual. So an implant is likely to be palatal to the position which would allow the most aesthetic replacement of the missing tooth.

There is a tendency, therefore, to place the crown onto the implant in a position that is labial to the implant ie the implant will overlap the labial border of the ridge.

Hence 'ridgelapping'

The danger of ridgelapping is that it is, in effect, a labial cantilever on the implant.

In this example, the most aesthetic placement of the crown is **labial** to the position of implant, which has been restricted by the resorption of the alveolus in a palatal direction.

This results in a cantilevered occlusal force on the implant and may also be associated with inflammation of the marginal gingivae.

This may be detrimental to the implant and cause failure.

| Ideal ridge form for the implant to support aesthetic crown |

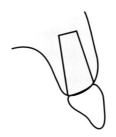

| Resorbed ridge form resulting in excessive ridgelapping (for aesthetic reasons) |

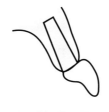

☐ Crown ☐ Bone ☐ Implant

sents a challenge, because the clinician has the opportunity to:

- Decide the size and shape of the occlusal table
- Choose the number, position, size and orientation of the implants
- Modify the quantity and architecture of the bone.

These variations are not, of course, without limit and there will be constraints imposed by the patient's condition. Nevertheless the many different types and designs of prostheses, the considerable number of available implant systems and the possibility of bone augmentation offer considerable choice for each and every case.

These choices can only be enjoyed by patients of those dentists who plan ahead.

This large number of variables that exists within these design options emphasise the need for careful treatment planning and *communication* within the treatment team (surgeon, restorative dentist, laboratory technician and maybe hygienist and/or general dental practi-

tioner). The process follows the previously described EDEC principle.

Presented below are some of the variables and their relationship to occlusion.

1. Relationship between occlusal table and implant diameter

Cantilevered forces may result from extending the prostheses beyond where the implants are located or arise more subtly in the form of ridge-lapped fixed prostheses (Fig. 3). Both are a source of non-axial loading and, therefore, potentially risk implant failure. Clearly, the relationship between implant diameter and occlusal dimensions are linked to non-axial loading (Fig. 4 and 5a,b).[39–40] Non-axial loading is to be avoided if at all possible.

If the ridge is narrow, because of resorption, the solution may be:

- Not only a narrow implant, but also a narrow crown
- Bone augmentation or bone manipulation, to allow a wider implant to be inserted.

E = Examine
D = Design
E = Execute
C = Check

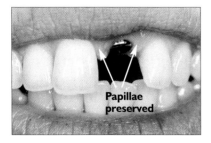
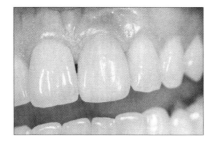

Fig. 4a-c If the implant is inserted before vertical bone loss has occurred, a normal clinical crown length will result (see Fig. 6a)

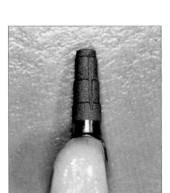

Fig. 5a Buccal view of failed implant that was supporting an occlusal table with a slight distal cantilever

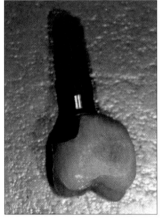

Fig. 5b Distal view of the same implant supporting crown with excessive buccal cantilever. Unsurprisingly this implant dramatically failed.

2. Ideal occlusal morphology

Provide an occlusion which is:

- Balanced occlusion with low cuspal angles and freedom in centric occlusion[41]
- Complimentary to the existing occlusion
- Achievable (lingualised occlusion may be easiest)
- Free of any non-axial forces (ie no inclined contacts and posterior interferences).

3. The significance of implant length-crown length ratio

In simple terms, a crown length to implant length ratio of 1:2 is ideal. To achieve this, early implant placement before vertical bone height has been lost is recommended. Immediate, or delayed implant insertion (at 6 to 12 weeks after extraction in the absence of bone pathology) usually facilitates the optimal crown/implant ratio. In practice, this means that the implant option needs to be considered before the extraction of a tooth.

With increasing vertical bone loss the implant-crown ratio will become progressively less favourable (Fig. 6a-c), not just in terms of loading but also in terms of aesthetic results and hygiene maintenance. Once the implant-crown ratio approaches 1:1 a removable prosthesis should be considered. Although the relationship between the head of the implant and the occlusal plane has obvious loading implications which are likely to affect implant success rates, there are no published studies in this area.

Guideline: Maximise the implant to crown ratio when anatomically possible. With significant vertical bone loss, a fixed prosthesis may not be feasible unless pre-implant bone grafting is acceptable to re-establish favourable inter-arch vertical relationships.

4. The site and nature of the implant bed

It is known that for osseointegration to occur predictably certain conditions must be met:

- The implant must consist of a suitable biomaterial with appropriate surface properties
- Adequate vital bone must be present to support and integrate with the implant
- A precise surgical fit must be achieved between the bone and the implant

Clinical studies and experience have shown that implants placed into the posterior maxilla can be expected to show lower success rates,[19,42] this may be caused by the potentially higher occlusal loads at the back of the mouth. Equally, an implant site that has been augmented (regardless of the material or technique used) can be expected to possess a reduced ability initially to withstand occlusal load. This effect might be permanent or temporary, depending upon the material used and the ability of that material to bond with or become replaced by vital bone.

Guideline: The ability of the implant bed to support occlusal load is dependant upon:

- *Site (occlusal load potentially increases towards the back)*
- *Quality of supporting bone (stable autogenous bone with no augmentation is the 'gold standard').*

5. The importance of monitoring of occlusal load

Since osseointegrated implants cannot move by nature of their relationship with bone, there is a considerable temptation to consider that restored implants require little if any monitoring. However, the nature of occlusal contacts and relationships can change as a result of many fac-

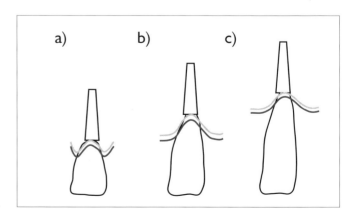

Fig. 6a-c Illustration of how the implant to crown ratio becomes progressively worse (loading and aesthetics) with increasing vertical bone loss. (Yellow line is the bone level and the red line is the gingival margin)

Summary of occlusal guidelines:

- **Select the widest diameter implant**
- **Provide a vertical emergence profile with no ridge lapping to avoid non-axial loading**
- **In narrow ridges consider a removable prosthesis, ridge augmentation, or abandoning implant treatment**
- **The occlusal table should be designed not to overload the bone-implant interface**

tors including tooth and prosthesis wear (Fig. 7), loss of teeth or implants, and mucosal atrophy.[43]

Guideline: Regularly evaluate the occlusal relationships of the implant supported prosthesis (at short intervals, typically 3–6 months). The provision of any treatment that has the potential to change the occlusion anywhere in the mouth should be the trigger to check the occlusion of an implant supported prosthesis. Accurate occlusal records of the starting point are extremely helpful.

Pre-treatment examination and case 'work up'

Not all cases will need all of the stages laid out below. These stages are presented as guidelines to ensure that the occlusion provided by a prosthesis supported by implants is well tolerated by the patient.

Examination

A short examination of the patient's articulatory system (TMJ, Muscles, Occlusion) is needed to diagnose any pre-existing TMD . This will include any signs of an active parafunction (tongue scalloping and cheek ridging). In particular, a note would be made of any evidence that occlusal factors contributed to the loss of teeth for which implant treatment is being considered. This could alter the treatment plan considerably.

A qualitative and quantitative assessment of the potential implant bed will influence the type of the prosthesis and the occlusal table that it can provide.

Case 'work up'

Study models mounted on a semi-adjustable articulator after facebow record will make it much simpler to examine the existing occlusion and to design an appropriate occlusal scheme

A *diagnostic wax-up* or pre-implant diagnostic prosthesis will help the restorative clinician and the laboratory technician plan the eventual prosthesis. It will also be an aid in the construction of any temporary or provisional restorations.

A *surgical stent* is a device that enable the ideal position of the implants to be visualised at the surgical phase of treatment. Its use is more than simply a surgical aid, it embodies the principle that the position of the implants should (within the physical constraints of the alveolar bed) be determined by the aesthetic and occlusal objectives of the final restorations. A diagnostic wax up (see section on Good Occlusal Practice in Advanced Restorative Dentistry) will greatly facilitate the construction of a useful surgical splint. The principle that the position of the implants will be determined before the surgical appointment and by factors including the aesthetic and occlusal objectives of the treatment plan is paramount.

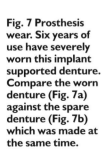

Fig. 7 Prosthesis wear. Six years of use have severely worn this implant supported denture. Compare the worn denture (Fig. 7a) against the spare denture (Fig. 7b) which was made at the same time.

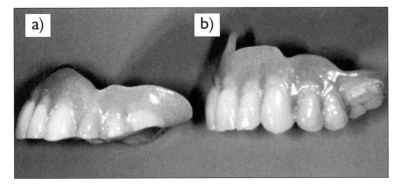

a)   b)

1. Buser D, Dula K, Belser U, Hirt H P, Berthold H. Localised ridge augmentation using guided bone regeneration 1. Surgical procedure in the maxilla. *Int J Period & Rest Dent* 1993; **13**: 29-45
2. Adell R, Lekholm U, Rockler B, Branemark P I. A 15-year study of osseointegrated implants in the treatment of the edentulous jaw. *Int J Oral Surg* 1981; **10**: 387-416.
3. Zarb G. Osseointegration: a requiem for the periodontal ligament? *Int J Period & Rest Dent* 1991; **11**: 88-91.
4. Weiner S, Klein M, Doyle J L, Brunner M. Identification of axons in the peri-implant region by immunohistochemistry. *Int J Oral Maxillofac Implants* 1995; **10**: 689-695.
5. Jacobs R, van Steenberghe D. Comparison between implant-supported prostheses and teeth regarding passive threshold level. *Int J Oral Maxillofac Implants* 1993; **8**: 549-554.
6. Hammerle C H, Wagner D, Bragger U *et al.* Threshold of tactile sensitivity perceived with dental endosseous implants and natural teeth. *Clin Oral Implants Res* 1995; **6**: 83-90.
7. Trulsson M, Gunne H S. Food-holding and biting behavior in human subjects lacking periodontal receptors. *J Dent Res* 1998; **77**: 574-582.
8. Rosen P S, Summers R, Mellado J R *et al.* The bone-added osteotome sinus floor elevation technique: multicenter retrospective report of consecutively treated patients. *Int J Oral Maxillofac Implants* 1999; **14**: 853-858.
9. Keller E E, Tolman D E, Eckert S E. Maxillary antral-nasal inlay autogenous bone graft reconstruction of compromised maxilla: a 12-year retrospective study. *Int J Oral Maxillofac Implants* 1999; **14**: 707-721.
10. Mericske-Stern R, Perren R, Raveh J. Life table analysis and clinical evaluation of oral implants supporting prostheses after resection of malignant tumors. *Int J Oral Maxillofac Implants* 1999; **14**: 673-680.
11. Lekholm U, Gunne J, Henry P, Higuchi K, Linden U, Bergstrom C, van Steenberghe D Int Survival of the Branemark implant in partially edentulous jaws: a 10-year prospective multicenter study. *J Oral Maxillofac Implants* 1999; **14**: 639-645.
12. Balshi T J, Wolfinger G J, Balshi S F. Second Analysis of 356 pterygomaxillary implants in edentulous arches for fixed prosthesis anchorage. *Int J Oral Maxillofac Implants* 1999; **14**: 398-406
13. Froum S J, Tarnow D P, Wallace S S, Rohrer M D, Cho S C. Sinus floor elevation using anorganic bovine bone matrix (OsteoGraf/N) with and without autogenous bone: a clinical, histologic, radiographic,

and histomorphometric analysis. Part 2 of an ongoing prospective study. *Int J Periodontics Restorative Dent* 1998; **18**: 528-543.

14. Ivanoff C J, Grondahl K, Sennerby L, Bergstrom C, Lekholm U. Influence of variations in implant diameters: a 3- to 5-year retrospective clinical report. *Int J Oral Maxillofac Implants* 1999; 14: 173-180.

15. Morris H F, Ochi S Hydroxyapatite-coated implants: a case for their use. *J Oral Maxillofac Surg* 1998; **56**: 1303-1311.

16. Karlsson U, Gotfredsen K, Olsson C A 2-year report on maxillary and mandibular fixed partial dentures supported by Astra Tech dental implants. A comparison of 2 implants with different surface textures. *Clin Oral Implants Res* 1998; 9: 235-242.

17. Watson R, Marinello C, Kjellman O, Rundcrantz T, Fahraeus J, Lithner B. Do healing abutments influence the outcome of implant treatment? A three-year multicenter study. *J Prosthet Dent* 1998; **80**: 193-198.

18. Albrektsson T, Zarb G A, Worthington P, Eriksson A R. The long-term efficacy of currently used dental implants: a review and proposed criteria of success. *Int J Oral Maxillofac Surg* 1986; **1**: 11-25.

19. Watson C J, Tinsley D, Ogden A R, Russell J L, Mulay S, Davison E M. A 3- to 4-year study of single tooth hydroxylapatite coated endosseous dental implants. *Br Dent J* 1999; 187: 90-94.

20. Preiskel H W, Tsolka P. Treatment outcomes in implant therapy: the influence of surgical and prosthodontic experience. *Int J Prosthodont* 1995; **8**: 273-279.

21. Weyant R J. The case for clinical registries. *In* Trotman C A, McNamara J A. (eds) *Orthodontic treatment: outcome and effectiveness.* 1st ed pp 319-343. Ann Arbor: University of Michigan.

22. el Askary AS, Meffert RM, Griffin T Why do dental implants fail? Part I. *Implant Dent* 1999; **8**: 173-185.

23. Esposito M, Lausmaa J, Hirsch J M, Thomsen P. Surface analysis of failed oral titanium implants. *J Biomed Mater Res* 1999; 48: 559-568.

24. Esposito M, Thomsen P, Ericson L E, Lekholm U. Histopathologic observations on early oral implant failures. *Int J Oral Maxillofac Implants* 1999; 14: 798-810.

25. O'Mahony A, Spencer P Osseointegrated implant failures. *J Ir Dent Assoc* 1999; 45: 44-51.

26. Newman 1988 Newman MJ, Flemmig FT. Periodontal considerations of implants and implant associated microbiota. *J Dent Educ* 1988; **52**: 737.

27. Esposito M, Hirsch J, Lekholm U, Thomsen P. Differential diagnosis and treatment strategies for biologic complications and failing oral implants: a review of the literature. *Int J Oral Maxillofac Implants* 1999; **14** : 473-490.

28. Isidor F. Histological evaluation of peri-implant bone at implants subjected to occlusal overload or plaque accumulation. *Clin Oral Implants Res* 1997; 8: 1-9.

29. Palmer R, Palmer P, Howe L. Dental implants: Part 10. Complications and maintenance. *Br Dent J* 1999: **187**: 653-658.

30. M Norton. Fixed bridge rehabilitation. *In* M.Norton *Dental Implants: a guide for the general practitioner.* 1st ed. pp 81-104. London: Quintessence Publishing Co Ltd,1995.

31. Muftu A, Chapman R J. Replacing posterior teeth with freestanding implants: four-year prosthodontic results of a prospective study. *J Am Dent Assoc* 1998; **129** : 1097-1102.

32. Bahat O, Handelsman M. Use of wide implants and double implants in the posterior jaw: a clinical report. *Int J Oral Maxillofac Implants* 1996; 11: 379-386.

33. Balshi T J, Hernandez R E, Pryszlak M C, Rangert B A comparative study of one implant versus two replacing a single molar. *Int J Oral Maxillofac Implants* 1996; **11**: 372-378.

34. Schwartz-Arad D, Samet N. Single tooth replacement of missing molars: a retrospective study of 78 implants. *J Periodontol* 1999; 70: 449-454.

35. Reitz J V. Lingualized occlusion in implant dentistry. *Quintessence Int* 1994; **25**: 177-180.

36. Rodriguez A M, Aquilino S A, Lund P S, Ryther J S, Southard T E. Evaluation of strain at the terminal abutment site of a fixed mandibular implant prosthesis during cantilever loading. *J Prosthodont* 1993 ; **2**: 93-102.

37. Chapman R J, Kirsch A Variations in occlusal forces with a resilient internal implant shock absorber. *Int J Oral Maxillofac Implants* 1990; **5**: 369-374.

38. Garcia L T, Oesterle L J. Natural tooth intrusion phenomenon with implants: a survey. *Int J Oral Maxillofac Implants* 1998; 13: 227-231.

39. Weinberg L A, Kruger B. An evaluation of torque (moment) on implant/prosthesis with staggered buccal and lingual offset. *Int J Periodont Restor Dent* 1996; **16**: 252-265.

40. Weinberg L A Reduction of implant loading using a modified centric occlusal anatomy. *Int J Prosthodont* 1998; 11: 55-69.

41. Kaukinen J A, Edge M J, Lang B R. The influence of occlusal design on simulated masticatory forces transferred to implant-retained prostheses and supporting bone. *J Prosthet Dent* 1996; **76**: 50-55.

42. Jaffin R A, Berman C L. The excessive loss of Branemark implants in type IV bone: a 5-year analysis. *J Periodontol* 1991; **62**: 2-4.

43. Dario L J. How occlusal forces change in implant patients: a clinical research report. *J Am Dent Assoc* 1995; **126**: 1130-1133.

The completed list of the guidelines of good occlusal practice

1   The examination of the patient involves the teeth, periodontal tissues and articulatory system.
2   There is no such thing as an intrinsically bad occlusal contact, only an intolerable number of times to parafunction on it.
3   The patient's occlusion should be recorded, before any treatment is started.
4   Compare the patient's occlusion against the benchmark of ideal occlusion.
5   A simple, two dimensional means of recording the patient's occlusion before, during and after treatment is an aid to good occlusal practice.
6   The conformative approach is the safest way of ensuring that the occlusion of a restoration does not have potentially harmful consequences.
7   Ensuring that the occlusion conforms (to the patient's pre-treatment state) is a product of examination, design, execution and checking (EDEC)
8   The 'reorganised approach' involves firstly the establishment of a 'more ideal' occlusion in the patient's pretreatment teeth or provisional restorations; and then adhering to that design using the techniques of the 'conformative approach'
9.   An 'ideal occlusion' in removable prosthodontics is one which reduced de-stabilising forces
10.   The occlusal objective of orthodontic treatment is not clear, but a large discrepancy between centric occlusion and centric relation should not be an outcome of treatment
11.   An 'orthodontic' examination of the occlusion should include: the dynamic occlusion; and the jaw relationship in which the patient has centric occlusion
12.   The occlusion of periodontally compromised teeth should be designed to reduce the forces to be within the adaptive capabilities of the damaged periodontia
13.   Good occlusal practice in children is determined by the needs of the developing occlusion, consequentially 'restoration at all costs' may not be the best policy.
14.   Not all tooth surface loss needs treatment, but effective monitoring is essential
15.   Dento-alveolar compensation has often occured in patients exibiting marked tooth surface loss.
16.   The occlusal prescription of an implant supported restoration needs to take account of the features of osseointegration
17.   The occlusion should be planned before implants are placed

Index